P9-BIL-935

101 WAYS TO LOWER YOUR CHOLESTEROL

Easy Tips That Allow You to
Take Control, Reduce Risk, and Live Longer

SHIRLEY S. ARCHER with DAVID EDELBERG, MD

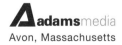

Aadamsmedia
Avon, Massachusetts

Contains material adapted and abridged from *The Everything® Low Cholesterol Book*
by Shirley Archer, copyright © 2004 by F+W Media, Inc.,
ISBN 10: 1-59337-146-2, ISBN 13: 978-1-59337-146-3.

Published by
Adams Media, a division of F+W Media, Inc.
57 Littlefield Street, Avon, MA 02322. U.S.A.
www.adamsmedia.com

ISBN 10: 1-60550-129-8
ISBN 13: 978-1-60550-129-1

Printed in the United States of America.

10 9 8 7 6 5 4 3 2 1

Library of Congress Cataloging-in-Publication Data
is available from the publisher.

This book is available at quantity discounts for bulk purchases.
For information, please call 1-800-289-0963.

Contents

The Big Picture of Cholesterol Health

Cholesterol may not seem like the most exciting topic in the world, but given the huge role it plays in your health, cholesterol is actually very important. You've probably heard about it in the news, seen it on nutrition labels, or even had a discussion about it during a visit to your doctor's office. While cholesterol is a naturally occurring substance that appears in each cell in the body, it is also something that can get out of control if it's not properly monitored and managed. All kinds of things contribute to your cholesterol status, from what you eat and your level of physical activity to your family history and the condition of your overall health. This means that it often takes a multipronged approach to keep your cholesterol on track.

You've doubtless heard all sorts of scary statistics about the numbers of deaths due to heart attacks, strokes, and other heart-disease-related events. You've probably also heard that incidence of obesity and related conditions such as diabetes are on the rise in this country. While those statistics and numbers are factual, it doesn't mean that you, too, will become a statistic. That's why you've picked up this book, right? You've already begun to take the reins on your health in order to ensure a long, healthful future for yourself. This, in itself, is a big part of the battle.

Now that you have this book in hand, it's time to start delving into the deeper issues. In the following chapters you'll first learn what cholesterol is and how it works, and then you'll go on to find out how you can monitor and manage it with tests and treatments. You'll also read about changes you can make in your diet and lifestyle to keep yourself feeling good, inside and out. Part IV offers delicious and nutritious recipes that you can work into your meal plan, and Part V is all about weight management and exercise. In short, you've got all your bases covered. Just follow the advice in this book, and you'll be well on your way to a happier, healthier life.

PART I

WHAT IS CHOLESTEROL?

CHAPTER 1

The Basic Breakdown

Cholesterol is a waxy "lipid," or fatlike substance, that is a necessary and natural part of each cell in the body. It helps to maintain the structure of the walls of cell membranes, and it also works to keep our brains healthy. The liver manufactures cholesterol and uses it as raw material in the creation of important hormones and digestive enzymes. In addition to being manufactured in the body, cholesterol gets into the bloodstream through the food that you eat. In particular, if you eat too much saturated fat, the result is an elevated blood cholesterol level. The big picture, however, is not as simple as that. Many other factors play a role in the composition of cholesterol levels.

1. Learn How the System Works

The major players in the cholesterol picture are the liver and the blood fats. To support bodily functions, the liver synthesizes cholesterol, lipoproteins, triglycerides, and phospholipids. The liver manufactures both low-density and high-density lipoprotein (LDL and HDL) that are needed to transport cholesterol into the bloodstream for use in other tissues. The liver also collects them back from the bloodstream to keep blood cholesterol from getting too high. Blood fats are the building blocks the liver uses to produce cholesterol.

The body uses LDL cholesterol to build cell membranes, create essential hormones, and form digestive enzymes. This LDL cholesterol needs to be transported throughout the body. However, cholesterol is fatty and blood is watery; oil and water do not mix. This dilemma is resolved in the liver, where cholesterol is combined and coated with proteins to create lipoproteins. The protein coating enables fat to travel in the bloodstream.

To simplify how this process works, imagine a pickup and delivery service to and from the liver, which is the cholesterol manufacturing plant. Imagine that the lipoproteins are like delivery trucks that carry packages of cholesterol in the bloodstream. The function of the HDL "delivery trucks" is to pick up excess LDL cholesterol "packages" from the bloodstream and return them to the liver for repackaging as needed.

Another type of lipoprotein, VLDL, or very low-density lipoprotein, acts as the delivery truck that transports the LDL cholesterol throughout the body and delivers it to all the cells. The cell receptors are the dropoff stops where the LDL deliveries are made. The VLDL delivery truck also carries blood fats called triglycerides. These fats are available for immediate use by the body as energy, or for storage in fat cells for later use.

2. Don't Overload the System

Unfortunately, modern living conditions strain the system. By eating too much and moving too little, people make it all too easy for this delicately balanced delivery, pickup, and storage system to break down. The efficiency begins to fail when more LDL packages are transported in the bloodstream than are needed by the body's tissues. This excess LDL cholesterol continues to circulate in the bloodstream, increasing fat levels in the bloodstream and contributing to congestion on the "roadways" or arteries.

If this excess LDL occurs at the same time that too few HDL trucks are available to collect and deliver it back to the liver for recycling, then the LDL cholesterol starts to collect like piles of litter on the arterial walls in places where it finds areas of inflammation. Certain packages of this arterial litter become oxidized, and they begin the process that leads to the clogging up of the "roadways." Over time, this collection of debris on the arterial walls leads to a complete blockage, which then prevents blood flow that delivers essential oxygen for survival to the body's tissues. If this happens in the muscle tissues of the heart, the result is a heart attack that can lead to death.

The leading causes of the system breakdown are the following:

- **Overproduction of LDL packages.** The liver produces too much LDL cholesterol for the body's needs and much more than the HDLs can pick up.

- **Fleet reduction of HDL pickup trucks.** The liver does not produce or release enough HDLs into the bloodstream to pick up the excess LDLs.
- **Breakdown of liver management dispatch system.** The liver does not correctly signal to the body that it needs to pick up more LDLs.
- **Damage to roadways.** Inflammation is present in the interior walls of the arteries.
- **Transformation of LDL packages into litter.** Free radicals (independent and unstable oxygen molecules in the body) attach to certain LDL packages and "oxidize" them, causing them to become large and sticky and attach to blood vessel walls.

Research suggests that there are seven LDL subtypes and five HDL subtypes. Some of these subtypes are more harmful and others are more beneficial to health. For LDL cholesterol, particle size plays a significant role in the risk picture. People with higher numbers of the small dense LDL particles, rather than the large fluffy LDL particles, have a significantly higher risk of heart attack.

Plaque is another detail of this picture. Plaque is composed of oxidized LDLs and calcium in the bloodstream, as well as other cellular debris, or litter, that gets caught in the fatty (lipid) deposits. As the deposit grows larger, it hardens from the increase in the amount of calcium. Plaque is living and growing. It has an outer layer of scar tissue that covers the calcium and fats, as well as the white blood cells that responded to the damaged arterial wall within. Eventually the buildup of plaque can decrease or block blood flow to the heart or to the brain, starving these organs of essential oxygen and causing chest pains, a heart attack, or a stroke. This plaque buildup is known as atherosclerosis and is one of the most common types of heart disease.

3. Know the Good, the Bad, and the Ugly

The various types of lipoproteins are outlined in the following chart:

Types of Lipoproteins

Name	Type of Lipoprotein	Nickname
HDL	High-density lipoprotein	"Good" cholesterol
LDL	Low-density lipoprotein	"Bad" cholesterol
VLDL	Very low-density lipoprotein	
SDLDL	Small, dense, low-density lipoprotein	
Lp(a)	Apoliprotein (a) plus low-density lipoprotein	"Ugly" cholesterol

HDL Cholesterol

High-density lipoprotein (HDL) cholesterol, or the pickup truck fleet, is known as the "good" cholesterol. HDLs are considered "good" because they help clear the excess LDL cholesterol from your arteries. For a healthy heart and circulatory system, your HDL cholesterol levels should be higher than 40 mg/dL. The higher the level of your HDLs, the better it is for your health. People who have low levels of HDL cholesterol are at higher risk for heart disease.

According to the National Cholesterol Education Program (NCEP) guidelines, an HDL level of 60 mg/dL is considered a negative risk factor. A negative risk factor is like a bonus point that can negate or counteract another risk factor (such as having excess weight) when you are calculating your total risk score.

LDL Cholesterol

Low-density lipoprotein (LDL) cholesterol is known as the "bad" cholesterol; however, LDL cholesterol is bad for your body only if you have too much in your bloodstream or you have too much of the particularly harmful subtype. LDL cholesterol is an essential building block for cell membranes and is the substance from which hormones, including cortisol and testosterone, are manufactured. The amount of LDL cholesterol that exceeds what your body needs, however, flows through your bloodstream and increases the likelihood of the formation of plaque that can block blood flow.

NCEP guidelines recommend that near-optimal levels for LDL are under 130 mg/dL. If you are at risk for heart disease because of other risk factors, then the recommended level for LDL is under 100 mg/dL. If you are at "very high" risk, the guidelines recommend aggressively lowering LDL to less than 70 mg/dL.

just the facts

Cholesterol and other fats are measured in milligrams per deciliter (mg/dL). Some European labs use a measuring system of millimoles per liter (mmol/L). To convert millimoles to deciliters, multiply the mmol/L figure by 38.67.

Triglycerides (TRGs)

Triglycerides, or TRGs, are another type of fat that circulates in your bloodstream in the same way as HDL and LDL cholesterol. TRGs are composed of a sticky substance (called glycerol) and fatty acids. They can provide your body with a source of energy if needed. Triglyceride levels spike immediately after you eat and decrease slowly as the body processes nutrients from food that has been consumed. If muscles are working and active, the triglycerides can provide needed fuel. If the muscle cells do not use the circulating triglycerides to create energy, the TRGs are eventually deposited in the body's fat stores.

Since eating affects TRG levels, you should fast for at least nine to twelve hours before you have a lipid profile test. After you undertake this nine- to twelve-hour period without eating or drinking, the levels of TRG that are circulating in your bloodstream will more accurately reflect how much of these fats are consistently present in your blood.

A desirable level of TRG is less than 150 mg/dL. People who are overweight, who drink alcohol excessively, who are diabetic, or who have other disorders are prone to have elevated triglyceride levels. Women tend to have higher triglyceride levels than men.

Evidence from research shows that the risk of heart disease increases when the triglyceride level is too high, particularly when a person simultaneously has low levels of HDL cholesterol. Triglyceride levels of 500 mg/dL or above are associated with the risk of pancreatitis, which can lead to pancreatic cancer. Treatment is indicated for triglyceride levels above 150 mg/dL.

4. Evaluate Your Total Cholesterol

Total cholesterol is the sum total of all the cholesterol in your bloodstream at a given time. Different types of cholesterol, such as HDLs and LDLs, make up the total amount. Several factors affect the total cholesterol levels in your bloodstream, including:

- **Your diet:** Foods that come from animals, such as meats and eggs, contain cholesterol. Foods high in saturated fats, such as meats and dairy products, are converted into cholesterol in your body. Processed foods that contain trans fats are converted into LDL or "bad" cholesterol.
- **Your weight:** Excess consumption of dietary fat can lead to elevated cholesterol levels. People who lose as little as 10 percent of their total body weight have seen improvements in cholesterol levels.
- **Whether you smoke:** Smoking lowers levels of HDL, or "good" cholesterol. Two other heart disease risks are incurred by smoking: First, smoking increases the amount of free radicals in your body. These are altered oxygen molecules that can cause the LDL to precipitate into the lining of your blood vessels. Second, smoking increases the inflammation of the arteries, the piles of litter referred to earlier.
- **Whether you consume alcohol:** For some people, moderate alcohol consumption raises levels of HDL, or good cholesterol. Excess consumption is, of course, not healthful.
- **Your level of physical activity:** People who are physically active on a regular basis have higher levels of HDL, or good cholesterol. Inactivity leads to a relative increase in LDL, or bad cholesterol levels.
- **Whether you effectively manage stress:** Research studies show that mental and emotional stress can adversely affect heart health.

- **Your family history:** Familial hypercholesterolemia strikes one in 500 children. The strongest risk factor for heart disease is hereditary. If a family member has had a heart attack or stroke before the age of fifty-five, your odds of having heart disease are much greater.
- **Your gender and age:** Before menopause, women have a natural advantage over men as female hormones help to maintain high levels of HDL. As the body grows older, the risk of heart disease increases, though it typically takes years to develop to a life-threatening stage.
- **Your general state of health:** Several of the risk factors for heart disease are directly related to lifestyle habits that can be changed.

According to NCEP guidelines issued by the federal government and supported by leading researchers and the American Heart Association (AHA), desirable total cholesterol results should be lower than 200 mg/dL. Levels from 200 to 239 mg/dL are considered borderline high. Total cholesterol levels of 240 mg/dL and above are considered high.

CHAPTER 2

Cholesterol and Heart Disease

A healthy heart and circulatory system are something that many people take for granted—that is, until the day they experience chest pains or breathlessness and realize that something in the body is no longer working the way that it should. But what keeps a heart healthy? Or, what causes a heart to lose its ability to function properly? You'll find the answers to these and other questions in this chapter. Understanding what heart disease is and how cholesterol contributes to it is an important first step toward securing your health.

5. Learn the Structure and Function of the Heart

The human heart lies in the upper left center of the chest, next to the lungs. It has four chambers: the right atrium and the left atrium on the top, and the right and left ventricles on the bottom. Blood flows into the right side of the heart and out of the left side. To guide the flow of blood in one constant direction, each chamber connects to the next one through valves that open when the heart contracts.

---

did you know . . . ?

The circulatory system includes the heart, lungs, and all of the blood vessels. In the average person, these vessels would be 100,000 miles long if laid end-to-end. The heart pumps blood through these vessels to deliver oxygen and nutrients throughout the body and to remove carbon dioxide and other cellular waste products.

Blood that no longer contains oxygen enters the right side of the heart through a large vein called the vena cava. This deoxygenated blood flows into the right atrium. When the heart contracts, this blood flows through the tricuspid valve into the right ventricle. From the right ventricle, the blood enters the pulmonary artery via the pulmonary valve to become freshly oxygenated in the lungs. The newly oxygen-rich blood leaves the lungs and flows back to the heart's left atrium through the pulmonary vein. With the next contraction, the mitral valve opens and blood flows into the left ventricle, the strongest section of this miraculous muscular pump. When this section contracts, blood then rushes through the aortic valve into the aorta to repeat its journey around the body. This circulatory process continues automatically for as long as you live.

An electrical stimulus regulates the heartbeat. In the right atrium, a specialized group of cells—known as the sinoatrial node, the SA node, or the sinus node—triggers the electrical impulses that cause the chambers of the heart to contract and push the blood along its path. The rate of the electrical impulses is regulated, but it can vary depending on different chemical stimulators in the body. In this manner, a healthy heart can respond to different needs as required by the demands of life.

did you know . . . ?

A healthy heart is an electronically regulated muscular pump that is about the size of a fist. Each day and night, the average heart beats approximately 100,000 times and pumps 2,000 gallons of blood. Over a normal lifespan, the heart will beat more than 2.5 billion times.

The function of the heart and the circulatory system is to keep blood flowing continuously at a consistent rate. This ensures delivery of essential oxygen and nutrients to the body's tissues. Other processes that occur simultaneously through the circulation include the removal of waste products from cells back to the lungs, liver, and kidneys for filtering. A healthy nervous system is also important to a healthy circulatory system, since it affects heart rate and vessel function.

6. Understand Potential Heart Problems

Unfortunately, the heart doesn't always function perfectly. To comprehend the role of cholesterol and the process of atherosclerosis, and their impact on heart diseases, you need to be able to understand them in the context of the range of potential heart problems. There are several disorders that can have a negative effect on the circulatory process by reducing blood flow. Some of these disorders are genetic; others are either caused by or worsened by atherosclerosis, which can result from the presence of harmful types of cholesterol circulating in the bloodstream. The most common disorders are these:

- Arrhythmias, or malfunctions of the electrical system
- Congestive heart failure, or weakness of the muscular pump
- Congenital defects, such as a hole between the two atrial chambers (an atrial septal defect)
- Narrowing of the heart valves from calcification (stenosis) or from tumors in the heart
- Leaking valves, known as insufficiency, such as mitral valve prolapse
- Damage to the heart muscle itself from blockage of coronary arteries due to atherosclerosis

Each of these disorders results in a heart muscle that is not capable of pumping blood sufficiently. Atherosclerosis is the most common indirect factor in arrhythmia and congestive heart failure and a direct factor in block-age of coronary arteries.

7. Get Educated about Heart Attacks

When circulatory disorders impair blood flow to the heart muscle itself, a per-son experiences mild to severe chest pain. This chest pain can develop into a full-blown heart attack. The odds of a heart attack occurring are high. Since a person with heart disease may have no external symptoms prior to a heart attack, it is important to be aware of the warning signs.

Warning signs of a heart attack include the following:

- Uncomfortable pressure, fullness, squeezing, or pain in the center of your chest that lasts for more than a few minutes, or that recurs
- Pain that spreads from the chest to the shoulders, neck, jaw, or arms
- Chest discomfort combined with lightheadedness, fainting, sweating, nausea, or shortness of breath

If these symptoms come and go, and are generally triggered by exertion (such as stair-climbing, shoveling snow) and ease up with stopping the activ-ity, the situation is referred to as coronary insufficiency or angina pectoris. This could lead to a full-blown heart attack at some point, so make sure that you contact your doctor immediately for further testing.

Symptoms may range from severe to mild, or they may gradually worsen. For some people, symptoms come and go. The following are less common warning signs of a heart attack:

- Atypical (unusual) chest, stomach, or abdominal pain
- Nausea or dizziness
- Shortness of breath followed by difficult breathing
- Unexplained anxiety, weakness, or fatigue
- Heart palpitations, accompanied by a cold sweat or pale skin

If you experience any signs or symptoms of a heart attack, do not hesitate. Get medical help immediately. Every minute is important in a heart attack situation. Always keep emergency phone numbers in a convenient location near the telephone so no time will be wasted. Call 911 or your local emergency medical service (EMS) for an ambulance to take you to the hospital. While you are waiting for the ambulance, chew a couple of aspirin tablets. These will help dissolve any clot that is forming. Medical treatment, including clot-dissolving medicine, can save your life and reduce damage to the heart muscle, but only if treatment begins very soon after a heart attack occurs.

8. Know the Cholesterol/Heart Disease Connection

All heart diseases are referred to as cardiovascular diseases (CVDs). CVDs include high blood pressure, coronary heart disease, congestive heart failure, stroke, rheumatic heart disease, artery diseases, pulmonary heart disease, and congenital cardiovascular defects.

Coronary heart disease, also referred to as coronary artery disease (CAD), is the most common form and represents 54 percent of all CVDs. CAD includes angina pectoris, which is chest pain from narrowing of blood vessels, and myocardial infarction (MI), also known as a heart attack, from the complete blockage of blood supply to the heart.

It is possible for a person to have more than one type of CVD at the same time. For example, a person may have both CAD and high blood pressure. CAD is responsible for more than half of all cardiac events in men and women under age seventy-five. According to the National Heart, Lung, and Blood Institute's Framingham Heart Study, the lifetime risk of developing CAD after age forty is 49 percent for men and 32 percent for women.

Scientists now know that atherosclerosis can start in childhood. Researchers have found the beginning of fatty streaks in the arteries of children as young as three years old. The average American has significant buildup in his or her arterial walls by middle age. In women, possibly because of the protective effects of estrogen, the thicker buildups do not begin to show up until after menopause.

Even without the impact of a stroke or heart attack, atherosclerosis advances the aging process. Healthy circulation in the body is the source of nutrition and life for the cells. As this circulation is slowly cut off, it impairs the functioning of your cells. Atherosclerosis does not need to be inevitable. With knowledge of the mechanisms that contribute to this disease, you can take steps to reduce your risks and to prolong your youthful vitality and energy.

9. Take Your Health by the Horns

Whether you are young or old, male or female, you can improve your health and reduce your risk of CVDs by consistently monitoring and managing your cholesterol levels. While you cannot alter your heredity, you can make lifestyle changes that significantly lower risks, regardless of your genetic heritage. Even if you already have CAD, you can reap benefits by managing your cholesterol levels. Research evidence shows that decreasing your blood cholesterol levels can slow, stop, and even reverse plaque buildup over time. As you lower your LDL cholesterol levels and increase your HDL levels, you can reduce the cholesterol content in the unstable plaque that has built up in the arterial walls. Accordingly, you will reduce your future risks of having a heart attack.

Through effective cholesterol management, you can cut your risks of having a future heart attack and may even add valuable years to your life. At the same time, beyond extending your longevity, improving your lifestyle habits can also enrich the quality of those additional years of living. It is possible to become even healthier as you age; suffering years of disease, disability, and loss of vitality is not anyone's necessary fate. Adopting healthy habits extends your youthfulness and enhances your feelings of well-being. CVDs do not have to be such fearful killers. You can make a difference to improve your odds and to get even more enjoyment out of life.

CHAPTER 3

Risk Factors

Heart disease is a multifactorial disease, meaning that multiple factors contribute to the development and progression of the disease. One risk characteristic alone, such as age, is generally not enough to trigger the disease. However, a combination of factors, such as age, inactivity, smoking, and improper nutrition, can easily support the progression of heart disease over time. The more risk factors that you possess, the greater your likelihood of having the disease. Fewer risk factors, on the other hand, mean less likelihood of having the disease.

10. Identify Risk Factors

Any condition that indicates the presence of atherosclerosis signifies a high risk of coronary artery disease (CAD). These conditions include symptomatic carotid artery disease, peripheral arterial disease, and abdominal aortic aneurysm. If you are concerned about these, check with your doctor for more information. Researchers today also identify diabetes as a condition that creates a high risk of CAD. Diabetes is classified as carrying the equivalent risk of any of the other diseases that indicate the presence of heart disease.

Keep in mind that the basis for these risk factors is data from large population studies and is simply a reflection of profiles of those among the population who had a heart attack. Historically, however, research studies have not included in their database sufficient numbers of women, people from ethnic minorities, people from a variety of economic backgrounds, or people from a variety of lifestyles with different levels of access to health care. All of these factors, therefore, influence the applicability of these characteristic risk factors to any individual who may be different from those who have been studied.

The leading risk factors for heart disease are as follows:

- High total cholesterol and high LDL cholesterol
- Low HDL cholesterol
- Diabetes
- Cigarette smoking or inhaling secondary smoke
- Hypertension (high blood pressure)
- Unmanaged stress
- Physical inactivity or a sedentary lifestyle

- Excess weight
- Family history of heart disease
- Age and gender

This list includes several risk factors you can actively do something about. A few factors, such as your family history and your age and gender, are things you cannot change or control. The good news, however, is that you can make a strong impact on your modifiable risk factors. The way you choose to live your life every day plays a very important role in reducing your risk of heart disease. What you do makes a difference.

11. Understand Diabetes and the Metabolic Syndrome

Diabetes is a condition characterized by the failure of insulin to perform its normal functions. In a healthy body, the pancreas produces the hormone insulin and releases it into the bloodstream. The body uses this insulin to convert sugar, starches, and other foods into energy. When the system is not functioning normally, the bloodstream is overloaded with excess sugar. Genetics, excess weight, and inactivity all contribute to development of the disease.

Evidence from numerous research studies shows that people with diabetes mellitus have as much risk of having a heart attack as those who are already diagnosed with heart disease. To put this risk into statistical terms, people with diabetes have a 15 to 20 percent chance of having a heart attack within a ten-year period. This is the same level of risk as a person who is diagnosed with CAD. Furthermore, a person with diabetes has twice the likelihood of dying from a heart attack than a person who does not have diabetes.

just the facts

Because of the increased risk of heart disease associated with diabetes, the federal government guidelines recommend that people who are diabetic pursue the same cholesterol goals as those who have heart disease. Adults age forty-five and over should be tested to determine whether they are diabetic.

Researchers have identified a cluster of symptoms that includes abdominal obesity, high triglycerides, low HDL levels, high blood pressure, and a high fasting blood glucose level as contributors to a higher risk for heart disease. Studies have substantiated that individuals who have a cluster of three or more of these factors together have a greater risk of heart disease than someone who may only have one or two of the risk factors.

This clustering of several risk factors is described as the "metabolic syndrome." The reason for this reference is that the metabolic syndrome focuses on risk factors that have a metabolic origin. Carrying excess weight and leading an inactive lifestyle increase the likelihood of developing the metabolic syndrome. Medical experts agree that when an individual has diabetes or has the cluster of factors that make up the metabolic syndrome, he or she has a very high likelihood of having a heart attack. In addition to those conditions, there are several factors that can exacerbate the situation.

12. Stay Smoke-Free

Smoking is a risk factor because smokers have twice the risk of developing heart disease as nonsmokers in the same condition. Also, a smoker who has a heart attack is more likely to die from it than a nonsmoker. Cigarette smoking is the greatest risk factor for sudden cardiac deaths. Smoking low-tar or low-nicotine cigarettes does not make any difference in reducing your risk of heart disease. Nonsmokers who are frequently exposed to secondhand smoke also have an increased risk of developing heart disease.

Smoking contributes to heart disease because the chemicals that are inhaled from cigarette smoke reduce the amount of the good HDL cholesterol in your bloodstream. In addition, nicotine increases the rate of the heartbeat and constricts arteries, which leads to higher levels of blood pressure and stress on the heart and circulatory system. Some researchers believe that this can also lead to damage to arterial walls, making them more susceptible to plaque formation. Carbon monoxide reduces the amount of oxygen available to your body by up to 15 percent. Not only does this starve the body's tissue of essential oxygen, it also reduces the amount of oxygen being delivered to fuel the heart muscle. We constantly talk about "air pollution," yet one puff from a cigarette gives your lungs more pollution than any known air pollution "disaster" in history.

If you change this negative habit and quit smoking, you immediately begin to reduce your risk of heart disease. You also reduce your risks for lung cancer, lung disease, and other types of cancer. Your friends and loved ones reap the benefits of no longer being subject to secondhand smoke from you. Children raised in the homes of parents who smoke grow up with increased risks of developing asthma, lung cancer, and early heart disease.

13. Keep Tabs on Your Blood Pressure

High blood pressure occurs when the pressure of blood flowing through the blood vessels increases and remains elevated. This increase in pressure means that the blood flow is pushing against the arterial walls with a stronger than normal force. Over time, this increased pressure damages the arterial walls by causing them to become thicker and stiffer. The arterial walls lose elasticity. Research shows that damaged arterial walls are more likely to attract cholesterol and fats, which form plaque. This plaque formation leads to blockage of the arteries that can cause a heart attack or stroke.

did you know . . . ?

Blood pressure is measured in millimeters of mercury (mmHg) and consists of two numbers usually written one over the other. The top number reflects the systolic blood pressure reading—this is a measure of the pressure when your heart contracts, pumping the blood out. The bottom number reflects diastolic blood pressure. This reading measures the pressure when your heart rests, refilling with blood in between contractions.

In addition to contributing to arterial damage and consequent plaque formation, prolonged high blood pressure forces the heart to work harder and enlarge. Over time, the heart fails to function normally and cannot fully pump out all the blood it receives. This can cause fluids to back up into the lungs and can rob the rest of the body of the blood supply that it needs. This condition is known as congestive heart failure. If you have high blood pressure and you also have high cholesterol levels, your risk of having heart disease increases six times. If you have high blood pressure and high cholesterol levels and you are also a smoker, your risk of having heart disease increases by a factor of twenty.

Ideally, your blood pressure should be lower than 120 mmHg over 80 mmHg (usually spoken as "120 over 80" and written as 120/80). If either your systolic or your diastolic blood pressure reading is high, you may have high blood pressure. A high systolic blood pressure is a reading of 140 or above. A high diastolic blood pressure is a reading of 90 or above. It is important to pursue treatment if you have high blood pressure.

If high blood pressure is treated, the risk of heart disease and stroke is reduced. Blood pressure can be managed by losing as little as five to ten pounds of weight, exercising regularly, eating plenty of fruits, vegetables, and low-fat or nonfat dairy products, and reducing stress.

High blood pressure is dangerous because it usually gives no warning signs or symptoms. Doctors term high blood pressure "the silent killer." Be sure to get your blood pressure checked regularly, at least every two years. To determine whether or not you have high blood pressure, you will need to have it checked on several occasions and at different times of the day. Some people simply become nervous when they are in the doctor's office, resulting in a higher reading. Your blood pressure naturally changes during the day and rises dramatically when you are anxious. Make sure that you have multiple tests before you accept a diagnosis of high blood pressure.

14. Watch Your Weight and Get Active

Excess body weight is considered a risk factor because those who carry excess weight are at an increased risk of heart disease, high blood pressure, stroke, and diabetes, among other things. Carrying excess weight increases the strain on the heart and circulatory system, as well as on other body systems.

Just as the body needs a certain amount of LDL cholesterol to survive, it also needs a certain amount of body fat. However, excess body fat contributes to an increase in the natural production of higher levels of LDL cholesterol by the liver and to lower levels of HDL cholesterol. The delicate balance of the body's production and collection system of cholesterol becomes disturbed when the body carries additional fat stores. While the exact amount of fat that represents an excessive amount seems to vary from one individual to another, there generally seems to be a point at which too much body fat starts to harm, rather than to support, optimum health.

Conversely, when a person sheds excess body fat, the body's natural balancing mechanisms can begin to function effectively again. By losing excess fat, a person can stimulate the liver to decrease the production of LDL cholesterol and to increase the production of HDL cholesterol. This change can actually start to restore health to the circulatory system.

Inactivity is another big risk factor. People who are sedentary have twice the risk of heart disease as those who are active. The heart is a muscle. Like other muscles in the body, it becomes stronger with use. People are designed to be active, moving, living beings. Modern living conditions that include using cars and elevators, jobs that involve sitting at a desk working at a computer, and multiple other labor-saving devices have all but removed natural physical activity from our daily lives.

Adding some form of an endurance activity into your daily life conditions your heart, lungs, circulatory system, muscles, bones, brain, and nervous system. Being physically active reduces your risk of heart disease, and it reduces your risk of high blood pressure, diabetes, colon cancer, back pain, and cognitive disorders. Regular physical activity increases your levels of HDL or good cholesterol and lowers your level of total cholesterol.

The really great news is that research confirms that regular moderate-intensity exercise—at a minimum of thirty minutes a day on most days of the week—can have a powerful impact on improving your health. Moderate-intensity exercise includes activities like a brisk walk, fast enough that you break into a sweat but can still talk easily. To accumulate your thirty minutes of activity, you don't even have to do it all at once. People still enjoy improvements in health from as little as ten minutes of activity in three cumulative bouts over the course of the day.

PART II

CHOLESTEROL TESTING

CHAPTER 4

Know Your Numbers

Although cholesterol levels alone are not predictive of heart disease in all people, knowing your levels is a valuable first step toward understanding your risk status. When you know your cholesterol levels, as well as the status of your other risk factors, you gain valuable insight into the health of your current lifestyle. Furthermore, for those people who learn that they fall into high-risk categories, the sooner they begin a treatment plan, the sooner they can start to reduce their risks of heart attack or stroke.

15. Monitor Your Cholesterol Levels

A high total cholesterol level or a high LDL (bad) cholesterol level increases your risk of heart disease. As stated earlier in the book, a total cholesterol level is considered high if it is greater than 200 mg/dL.

According to the most recent government guidelines, ideal LDL cholesterol levels depend on how many other risk factors you have. For example, if you have one or no other risk factors, your LDL cholesterol level is considered high if it is greater than 160 mg/dL. It is considered "borderline high" if it is greater than 130 mg/dL. A total cholesterol greater than 240 mg/dL or an LDL cholesterol 160 mg/dL or greater are considered high risk.

If you have two or more risk factors (such as obesity, smoking, or inactivity), your LDL cholesterol level is considered high if it is equal to or greater than 130 mg/dL. If you have coronary artery disease (CAD) or an equivalent counterpart to other blood vessels (such as peripheral arterial disease, symptomatic carotid artery disease, or abdominal aortic aneurysm), your LDL cholesterol level is considered high if it is greater than 100 mg/dL.

If your total blood cholesterol is in the borderline-high or high category, you may be able to avoid medication if you make a real effort to change your diet and increase your activity levels to lower your cholesterol. If you succeed in lowering your cholesterol levels, you will definitely reduce your risk of heart disease. Virtually all coronary heart disease is caused by atherosclerosis, which occurs when cholesterol, fat, and other substances build up in the walls of the arteries that supply blood to the heart. Since atherosclerosis is a slow, progressive disease, you may not experience any symptoms for many years.

Lowering your total cholesterol level will slow plaque buildup in the arteries, may even reverse the plaque your body has already created, and reduce your risk of a future heart attack.

Low levels of HDL (good) cholesterol are considered a risk factor, since HDL cholesterol helps to prevent the buildup of cholesterol in the arteries. If you recall the liver manufacturing plant and the HDL pickup truck analogy from Chapter 1, you will remember that the HDL cholesterol gathers up free-floating cholesterol in the arteries and returns it to the liver. Low HDL levels mean there are fewer "trucks" available to clean up the arteries. An HDL cholesterol level of less than 40 mg/dL is considered low.

Two steps you can take to raise levels of HDL cholesterol are to increase physical activity levels to a minimum of thirty minutes on most days of the week and, if you smoke, to quit.

16. Follow Recommended Testing Schedules

Federal government guidelines recommend that all Americans check their cholesterol levels with a complete fasting lipoprotein profile at the age of twenty. The measurements taken by this test include your levels of total cholesterol, HDL cholesterol, LDL cholesterol, and triglycerides. If test results indicate that all levels are in a healthy range, then government guidelines recommend retesting at a minimum of five-year intervals. The full lipoprotein profile test is preferred over a test that only provides data regarding total cholesterol and HDL levels. Since diabetes is considered to carry a risk equivalent to that of heart disease, it is also a good idea to have your blood glucose levels checked.

just the facts

Evidence from research shows that atherosclerosis can start in childhood. If heart disease runs in the family, children should have their cholesterol levels checked regularly. In families that are high risk, it's even more important that from two years of age onward, children follow a healthy lifestyle that includes a nutritious low-fat diet and regular physical activity.

Although federal government guidelines recommend cholesterol testing for adults at least every five years, if you have had a major change of lifestyle during that five-year period, your cholesterol levels may be different and, therefore, worth checking again before five full years elapse. For example, if you were a college student at age twenty and then became a working professional after graduation at age twenty-one or twenty-two, your physical activity levels, dietary choices, and stress levels may have changed significantly. All of these factors can impact your cholesterol levels.

Under current government guidelines, if you fall into a category that requires treatment for your cholesterol levels, you will have your cholesterol tested at much more frequent intervals to evaluate the success of the treatment program and to make any necessary adjustments.

17. Consider Special Circumstances

Your general health also has an effect on your cholesterol test results. Do not go ahead with a scheduled cholesterol test if you have a cold or the flu.

Cholesterol levels drop temporarily during periods of acute illness, immediately following a heart attack or stroke, or during acute stressors such as surgery or an accident. For a more accurate measure, medical experts recommend that you wait at least six weeks after any illness before checking your cholesterol levels.

Your cholesterol levels reflect your lifestyle and your genetics. The ideal time to obtain an accurate test is when you are observing your usual routine. Cholesterol levels may change daily in response to deviations from your normal physical activity and eating habits, particularly if you increase your fat intake. Rapid weight loss also impacts cholesterol levels. These fluctuations in cholesterol do not occur immediately, but there is a definite response. Experts estimate that cholesterol levels may change by as much as 10 percent from one month to another simply from normal variations in metabolism. Therefore, for the truest insight into your risk of heart disease on the basis of your cholesterol levels, schedule your test at a time when you are living your typical, routine lifestyle.

During pregnancy, women's cholesterol levels typically escalate. Unless your health care provider advises you differently, an increase from your typical cholesterol levels at this time is not usually a cause for concern. Medical experts recommend that women wait at least until six weeks after delivery before checking cholesterol levels.

In some women, removal of the ovaries may trigger an increase in cholesterol levels. Menopausal women usually experience an increase in cholesterol levels that is thought to be related to reduced levels of estrogen. Be sure to discuss any changes in your typical cholesterol levels with your health care provider. Having an underfunctioning thyroid (hypothyroid) gland will cause your cholesterol to rise. If you have a family history of hypothyroidism and you are told your cholesterol is high, be sure to have your thyroid tested as well. In this situation, treating an underactive thyroid with thyroid hormone can dramatically lower levels of cholesterol.

Certain prescription medications may also lead to an increase in cholesterol levels. If you are taking any medications that have a potential adverse impact on your cholesterol levels, be sure that you understand how you will monitor your cholesterol levels over time to ensure that they remain within a healthy range.

18. Taking Your Blood Cholesterol Test

When you have your cholesterol tested, the test you should have is the full lipid profile. The results of this test include your levels of total cholesterol, HDL or good cholesterol, LDL or bad cholesterol, and triglycerides. For accurate results, you need to fast for nine to twelve hours before the test. That means you may have nothing to eat or drink but plain water during that time. It is important that you do not consume any alcoholic beverages, coffee, tea, or soda—only drink water.

What to Expect

Since you need to obtain a fasting profile, schedule your test for first thing in the morning. Your health care professional will take a blood sample, either from a vein or from a finger stick. After the health care provider has collected the blood, he or she may send it to a lab for analysis, or, if the test is being performed via a finger stick, a portable testing device will be used to analyze the sample.

If you are on any medications that affect cholesterol levels, work with your health care provider to determine whether you should not take your prescription for a certain period of time before you take your cholesterol test.

CHAPTER 5

Decoding Test Results

You've completed your cholesterol test, and you've received a report with various figures, a ratio, and maybe even a risk interpretation. But in addition to knowing your numbers, you also need to know what those numbers mean and whether you need to take action to change them. This chapter gives you insight into how to interpret your results in each of the following categories: total cholesterol, LDL cholesterol, HDL cholesterol, triglycerides, and ratio of total cholesterol to HDL cholesterol.

19. Understand Your Total Cholesterol Results

In general, the higher your total blood cholesterol level, the greater your risk of heart disease. For example, a person with a total cholesterol level of 240 mg/dL may have as much as twice the risk of heart disease as someone with a total cholesterol level of less than 200 mg/dL.

Total cholesterol alone, however, does not tell the complete story, because heart disease risk is related to the composition of your total cholesterol. For example, if you have high total cholesterol due to a very high HDL cholesterol level, then that is a positive condition. On the other hand, if your total cholesterol is not high, but you have a high LDL level or a low HDL level, then that is a negative condition.

Adults

The federal government and the American Heart Association recommend the following total cholesterol levels as a general guide for adults:

Classification of Total Cholesterol Levels for Adults

Total Cholesterol Level	Category
Less than 200 mg/dL	Desirable
200–239 mg/dL	Borderline high
240 mg/dL and above	High

If your levels fall into the "desirable" category of less than 200 mg/dL, the preliminary assessment of your heart attack risk is considered to be low, assuming that you do not have any other risk factors. Keep in mind, however, that as many as 50 percent of people who do not have elevated lipid levels, and who therefore fall within the "desirable" category, still have heart disease because of other risk factors.

Those who have cholesterol levels between 200 to 239 mg/dL are considered to be borderline high risk. This categorization, however, is not necessarily cause for alarm. If total cholesterol levels are high because of high HDL levels of more than 60 mg/dL, it actually means that you have a reduced risk of heart disease, assuming that you have no other risk factors.

People with total cholesterol levels of 240 mg/dL are classified as "high risk." More tests need to be undertaken without delay to develop a therapeutic treatment approach. People in this category are at higher risk of having a heart attack or stroke than those with normal levels.

Children and Adolescents

Scientific studies show that atherosclerosis actually begins in childhood. The federal government and the American Heart Association recommend the following guidelines on blood cholesterol in children and adolescents from the age of two to nineteen years:

Classification of Total Cholesterol Levels for Children and Adolescents

Total Cholesterol Level	Category
Less than 170 mg/dL	Acceptable
170–199 mg/dL	Borderline
200 mg/dL and above	High

Medical experts recommend cholesterol testing for children from families with a history of heart disease.

The majority of deaths from heart disease occur in older adults, simply because the disease has had more time to develop. Older adults include men age sixty-five years and older and women age seventy-five years and older. The challenge for older adults is that risk assessment by standard risk factors is less reliable, particularly as it is expressed as a percentage of risk over a ten-year period. This, however, does not mean that high total cholesterol levels in older adults should go untreated. Instead, we should keep in mind that elevated cholesterol levels in older adults simply do not have the same predictive power as they do for other adults.

20. Understand Your LDL Cholesterol Results

High levels of LDL cholesterol are known to be a major cause of heart disease. Federal government guidelines focus on reducing LDL levels as the primary means of providing therapy for people with high cholesterol. Strong research evidence supports the idea that reducing LDL levels results in reducing the risk of heart disease. However, before you assume that you have very high levels of LDL cholesterol based on the results of one test, make sure that you fasted for the recommended minimum of nine hours before you took your cholesterol test. If your LDL result was higher than 160 mg/dL and you are not certain you observed the fasting requirement closely, it's a good idea to repeat the test.

Adults

The following table reflects the classification of LDL cholesterol levels that are recommended by both the federal government and the American Heart Association for adults.

Classification of LDL Cholesterol Levels for Adults

LDL Cholesterol Levels	Category
Less than 100 mg/dL	Optimal
100–129 mg/dL	Near optimal
130–159 mg/dL	Borderline
160–189 mg/dL	High
Above 189 mg/dL	Very high

Current treatment approaches for people with high total cholesterol levels are based on LDL levels, the presence of other risk factors, and the calculated percentage of short-term risk of having heart disease.

People with elevated cholesterol levels are classified into four categories of risk for treatment. An existing diagnosis of CAD or an equivalent disease of the arteries or the presence of diabetes are very important factors that affect the treatment goal for LDL-lowering therapy. If the following conditions are present, the individual is considered to fall into the highest category of risk and is there-fore recommended to receive the most aggressive therapeutic treatment:

- Coronary artery disease
- Other forms of atherosclerosis, such as peripheral arterial disease, abdominal aortic aneurysm, and symptomatic carotid artery disease
- Diabetes
- Multiple risk factors that predict a ten-year risk of heart disease of greater than 20 percent

Children and Adolescents

Similar to the guidelines for total cholesterol, the recommended levels of LDL cholesterol in children differ slightly from the guidelines for adults. The following chart sets forth how various levels of LDL cholesterol are categorized in children:

Classification of LDL Cholesterol Levels for Children and Adolescents

LDL Cholesterol Levels	Category
Less than 110 mg/dL	Acceptable
110–129 mg/dL	Borderline
Above 129 mg/dL	High

For children, the government guidelines recommend lifestyle changes as the first line of therapeutic intervention. These changes include improving eating habits and increasing physical activity.

21. Understand Your HDL Cholesterol Results

Levels of HDL, or good cholesterol, show an inverse relationship to heart disease risk. Unlike LDL cholesterol and triglycerides, where high numbers mean increased risk, higher levels of HDL cholesterol mean a lower risk of heart disease. In healthy individuals, HDL cholesterol represents approximately 20 to 30 percent of total cholesterol levels.

The reasons for HDL cholesterol's beneficial effect are not exactly clear. Some researchers believe HDL cholesterol actively reverses atherosclerosis by carrying cholesterol away from arterial walls.

Some scientists believe that there may be multiple subtypes of HDL cholesterol, just as there are multiple subtypes of LDL cholesterol, and that some subtypes of HDL have more beneficial characteristics than others. These scientists believe that HDL2b, in particular, is important to the process of collecting excess LDL and returning it to the liver, thus maintaining healthy LDL levels.

Adults

A risk to health arises when HDL levels are too low. Evidence from studies shows that low HDL cholesterol is an independent risk factor for heart disease. This means that regardless of whether other risk factors are present, the risk of heart disease is higher for people with low HDL cholesterol. A 1 percent decrease in HDL levels is associated with a 2 to 3 percent increase in heart disease risk. The following chart sets forth the classification of HDL cholesterol levels as adopted by federal government guidelines and the American Heart Association:

Classification of HDL Cholesterol Levels for Adults

HDL Cholesterol Levels	Classification	Risk
Less than 40 mg/dL	Low HDL cholesterol	High risk
40–59 mg/dL	Moderate HDL cholesterol	Higher levels are desirable
60 mg/dL and above	High LDL cholesterol	Negative risk factor

Interestingly, adult women tend to have higher HDL cholesterol levels than adult men. According to government estimates, approximately one-third of all adult men and one-fifth of adult women have low HDL cholesterol levels that put them at increased risk of heart disease. At 40 mg/dL, however, both men and women can be considered to have low HDL—there is no separate recommendation for women. Nor is there a separate recommendation regarding HDL levels for children.

Natural strategies to increase HDL cholesterol include losing weight, increasing activity, and quitting smoking.

The Lipid Triad

Low HDL levels tend to occur in association with the presence of small, dense LDL particles (the worst type) and high levels of triglycerides. The relationship among these three types of lipids is known as the "lipid triad." Low HDL levels also tend to occur in conjunction with metabolic problems associated with insulin resistance. This condition, in which the body seems to "resist" the insulin's lowering effect on blood sugar, is considered to be a very early form of adult-onset diabetes. Therefore, many people who have the lipid triad also develop or already have Type 2 diabetes.

Several factors can lead to low HDL cholesterol levels. Many are variables related to lifestyle factors, and these can be changed by adopting healthy habits. People can raise their HDL by using diet changes to lower high triglycerides; reduce excess weight; increase physical activity; stop cigarette smoking; reduce high carbohydrate intake levels (more than 60 percent of total calories per day). In addition, drugs such as beta blockers, anabolic steroids, or progestational agents all affect HDL levels, as does heredity.

Approximately 50 percent of people who have low HDL levels have a genetic basis for their condition. Some of these people have a type of low HDL cholesterol known as "isolated low HDL," so called because it does not appear as part of the lipid triad. The other 50 percent of people, however, can change their HDL levels by improving their lifestyle habits.

High HDL: A Negative Risk Factor

Research shows evidence connecting high HDL cholesterol levels with a lower risk level for heart disease. For this reason, high HDL levels are considered a negative risk factor. The use of this terminology can be confusing. Risk factors are known to be those conditions that increase the level of risk for heart disease. So what does it mean for a risk factor to be negative?

What this term refers to is the fact that high HDL cholesterol is such a positive condition that it actually "negates" one of the other risk factors. If you think of a regular risk factor as adding points to your risk score, a negative risk factor is one that gives you negative points, or subtracts points from your score. For this reason, high HDL levels are very important for maintaining a healthy heart and circulatory system.

22. Understand Your Triglyceride Results

Triglycerides are a form of fat. They are present in most types of food and are the most common fat in the body. Triglycerides that float in the bloodstream provide fuel for energy. Those that are not used for fuel are stored in the body's fatty tissues. Recent research has made it clear that high triglyceride levels are a marker for increased risk of heart disease and are believed to be an independent risk factor. In addition, high triglycerides are usually present when other risk factors, such as diabetes and high LDL cholesterol, are present.

Adults

As the role of triglycerides in the process of developing heart disease becomes clearer, experts support efforts to keep triglyceride levels low. The federal government and the American Heart Association have come up with the following guidelines regarding fasting blood levels of triglycerides in adults:

Classifications of Triglyceride Levels for Adults

Triglyceride Levels	Classification
Less than 150 mg/dL	Normal
150–199 mg/dL	Borderline high
200–499 mg/dL	High
Above 499 mg/dL	Very high

As with low HDL cholesterol levels, both behavioral factors and genetics are the root causes of high triglyceride levels. Excess weight and lack of physical activity are the most common causes. However, any of the following can be a factor: cigarette smoking; excess alcohol consumption; very high carbohydrate intake levels (more than 60 percent of total calories per day); drugs such as beta blockers, corticosteroids, estrogens, and protease inhibitors for HIV; heredity; or other diseases such as Type 2 diabetes, chronic renal failure, and nephrotic syndrome. People who do not have any of these factors generally have triglyceride levels of less than 100 mg/dL. The first course of action to lower triglyceride levels is to adopt lifestyle changes, including improved nutrition and increased physical activity.

23. Understand Your Total Cholesterol and HDL Ratio

For a quick estimation of risk, you can calculate your total cholesterol and HDL ratio. To do this, divide your total cholesterol number by your HDL number. This method is based on the fact that high HDL levels relative to your total cholesterol are generally predictive of a lower risk of heart disease. While this estimate can give you a rough idea of your cholesterol level breakdown, it is not recommended as a test upon which to base therapeutic treatment.

Today, the American Heart Association recommends using absolute numbers for total blood cholesterol and HDL cholesterol levels. They are more useful to physicians than the cholesterol ratio in determining appropriate treatment for patients. If you're still interested in calculating your ratio, the classifications are as follows:

Classifications of Ratio of Total Cholesterol to HDL

TC/HDL Ratio	Classification
3.5 to 1	Optimum
4.5 to 1	Desirable
5 to 1 and above	High

To apply the formula, let's take an example of a woman with a total cholesterol level of 200 and an HDL level of 50. Her ratio is calculated by dividing 200 by 50, to equal a ratio of 4 to 1. According to this rough measure, her cholesterol is in the desirable range, but for a more comprehensive understanding, it's necessary to look at the entire spectrum of blood lipid levels.

CHAPTER 6

Diagnostic Tests and Other Markers of Heart Disease

Typically, your health care provider will include a cholesterol test as part of a routine physical checkup. In addition to blood lipid tests, medical professionals may use other tests to achieve a full picture of the health of the heart and circulatory system. This is particularly important if you have other risk factors, since 50 percent of people with "desirable" cholesterol levels still have heart disease.

24. Consider Noninvasive Diagnostic Tests

Several of the tests doctors use to measure the function of the heart and the state of the arteries are noninvasive, meaning that they are done without entering the body or puncturing the skin. Instead, medical professionals use different types of technology to look at the heart and arteries and to measure how well they are functioning. Some of these testing methods include:

- **Stress Test:** You exercise on a treadmill or a stationary bicycle to put your heart under stress. As you are exercising, medical professionals will administer tests to measure your heart's response to the stress. One such test is an electrocardiogram (EKG), which measures the electrical flow through your heart.

- **Echocardiogram:** An echocardiogram, also known as an "echo" test, uses sound waves to take a dynamic picture of the heart as it beats. A technician administers the test by placing a wand-like transducer on your ribs near the breastbone. This transducer transmits high-frequency sound waves directed toward the heart. The EKG machine receives electrical impulses that reflect the echoes of the sound waves and converts them into a dynamic picture of the heart. This reveals the shape and thickness of the walls in the heart's chambers and the large veins and arteries of the heart.

- **Cardiovascular Magnetic Resonance Imaging (MRI):** This test uses a magnet and radiofrequency waves to read signals from the body's cells to create an image of the interior of the body. MRI can provide detailed and accurate pictures of the size and thickness of the heart muscle, as well as data about the amount of blood flow. To take the test, the patient lies on a mobile examination table that moves through a large magnetic tube. The cardiologist analyzes the MRI images and data to evaluate the blood supply to the heart muscle and to assess the function of the blood vessels.

- **Ultrafast CT Scan or EBCT:** The ultrafast computerized tomography (CT) scan, also called electron beam computerized tomography (EBCT), is used to measure the amount of calcium deposited in your coronary arteries. The scanner is noninvasive and uses low-grade radiation to produce computer-generated pictures. With repeat evaluations, a cardiologist can track the rate of increase in calcification. This rate can provide further insight into the degree of risk of a heart attack.

25. Get Educated about Angiograms

An angiogram is an invasive test used to measure the degree of blockage in blood vessels. To perform an angiogram, the physician punctures a major artery and inserts a long plastic catheter up to a heart blood vessel. Then a dye known as a contrast agent is injected into the catheter to allow for observation of the heart blood vessels. The doctor observes the dye's progress on an X-ray machine to see how it flows through the vessels.

If the angiogram reveals a blockage, the doctor may perform an angioplasty, which involves clearing the blockage from the artery and then placing a hollow tube—called a stent—on the inside of the blood vessel to keep it open. If the blockage is so severe that the artery cannot be saved, bypass surgery may be required.

A challenge with angioplasty is that when the arterial blockage is cleared, it causes inflammation and swelling in the arterial walls, which can be just as obstructive as the plaque that had to be removed. This condition is called restenosis. Newer stents are drug-coated to prevent plaque from building back up into the artery or to keep tissue from growing into the inside of the stent.

26. Take a Blood Test for CRP

The presence of higher-than-normal levels of C-reactive protein (CRP) in the bloodstream is evidence of an infectious or inflammatory disease in the body. Medical professionals frequently give CRP tests to patients after surgery to determine whether an infection is present. Health care providers also use CRP tests to diagnose diseases, such as rheumatoid arthritis, and to evaluate the effectiveness of therapy. CRP is not indicative of the presence of a specific disease; it simply signals that the body is fighting some form of infection or inflammation.

Strong evidence from research studies shows that CRP is also a marker for heart disease. In the noteworthy Nurses' Health Study conducted by researchers from Brigham and Women's Hospital and from Harvard Medical School on 40,000 healthy, postmenopausal women, levels of CRP were clearly linked to heart disease risk. Women with high CRP levels were five times more likely than women with low CRP levels to develop heart disease and seven times more likely to have a stroke or heart attack.

The reason that CRP levels can be a marker for heart disease is related to the fact that damage to, or inflammation of, the interior lining of the arteries (referred to as the endothelial lining) precedes the formation of plaque. In other words, plaque collects in locations where there is damage to arterial walls. CRP can be evidence of this damage.

Given the strength of research evidence, some medical experts support the use of a high-sensitivity CRP (hs-CRP) test to measure the risk of a future heart attack or stroke. The value of the hs-CRP test is that it helps detect those individuals with low blood cholesterol levels who have high CRP levels and a high risk of heart attack. If you have low levels of CRP and healthy blood cholesterol levels, you can be that much surer that your risk of heart attack and stroke is really quite low. With a simple blood cholesterol test, you can be much less certain.

If you are fortunate enough to be able to get an hs-CRP test, be certain to take it when there are no other conditions that may increase the level of inflammation in your body. For example, do not take this test when you have any kind of infection, if you are injured, or if you know you are experiencing any type of inflammation.

Since their levels will already be elevated, people who suffer inflammatory-type conditions such as lupus or arthritis cannot use the hs-CRP test to accurately measure their risk for heart disease. The ideal candidate for an hs-CRP test is someone who is otherwise healthy, with healthy blood cholesterol levels, who is also concerned that he or she may be at risk for heart disease due to the presence of other risk factors.

Recently, doctors have made the correlation that people who do not take care of their gums (and who do not floss their teeth) regularly have a higher risk of developing heart disease. This has been explained by the chronic inflammation of the gums (gingivitis) that flossing prevents. If you learn that you have a high hs-CRP, schedule a visit to your dentist and get a status check on the health of your gums. You might be able to lower your hs-CRP and reduce your heart risks by flossing.

27. Consider an Lp(a) Blood Test

When LDL cholesterol combines with a substance known as apoliprotein (a), the result is a compound known as Lp(a), or "ugly" cholesterol. Evidence from some research studies shows that at high levels, it can increase a person's risk of heart attack or stroke, even if cholesterol levels are otherwise "desirable." Lp(a) is measured through a blood sample and can be tested as part of a lipoprotein panel.

just the facts

Approximately 50 percent of people who have heart attacks do not have elevated cholesterol levels. These individuals, however, typically have higher levels of CRP, Lp(a), apo B, or homocysteine.

Genetics determines your levels of Lp(a) and even the size of the Lp(a) molecule itself. Lifestyle changes do not alter levels of Lp(a); instead, levels for most people tend to remain consistent over a lifetime except for women, who will experience a slight rise in levels with menopause. Some physicians request testing of Lp(a) for patients who have a strong family history of premature heart disease or hypercholesterolemia. It can be a valuable test, particularly when other types of cholesterol are at healthy levels yet concern exists that heart disease is developing. Physicians will typically order this test if a patient has had a heart attack or stroke although cholesterol levels fall within a "healthy" category.

Treatment for elevated Lp(a) includes niacin therapy. Some experts believe that antioxidant therapy is also useful. People with high levels of Lp(a) benefit by concentrating their efforts on lowering LDL levels, since at lower levels it is harder for LDL particles to attach to plaque buildup. Lowering LDL levels ultimately lowers the level of risk.

28. Consider an Apoliprotein B (Apo B) Blood Test

Evidence from research shows that small, dense LDL is more highly associated with atherosclerosis than large, "fluffy" LDL. Studies also show that apoliprotein B (apo B) is a potential marker for the precise levels of LDL or bad cholesterol circulating in the bloodstream.

Apoliproteins are essential to the transport of blood lipids through the bloodstream and to the uptake of blood lipids into body cells. Apo B-100 is manufactured in the liver. It combines with very low-density lipoproteins (VLDL) to carry triglycerides and LDL cholesterol in the bloodstream. By measuring levels of apo B, it is possible to measure the exact number of LDL particles.

Some researchers believe that measurements of apo B may be better than LDL measurements when it comes to predicting the risk of heart disease. This is because levels of apo B can be measured directly, while LDL cholesterol levels are often calculated indirectly from levels of total cholesterol. These indirect calculations tend to be less accurate as triglyceride levels increase.

But experts believe that research evidence is not sufficient to support the superiority of apo B over LDL cholesterol measures. Therefore, federal government guidelines do not yet recommend the apo B measure as a factor in risk assessment. This may change as new tests continue to be developed and are more accurate and standardized.

29. Consider a Homocysteine Blood Test

Homocysteine is an amino acid and amino acids are the building blocks of proteins. Evidence from research studies shows that elevated levels of homocysteine in the blood are related to an increased risk of stroke, heart disease, and peripheral arterial disease. Blood levels of homocysteine escalate when the body lacks three B vitamins—folate, B_6, and B_{12}—that are essential to protein metabolism. Kidney disease can also lead to high homocysteine levels. Researchers continue to investigate the exact reason that elevated levels of homocysteine are related to vascular problems.

Some researchers theorize that increased levels of homocysteine damage the endothelial lining within the blood vessels. This damage creates the conditions for cholesterol to build up into plaque. Homocysteine also contributes to plaque ruptures, which can lead to harmful blood clot formation.

Homocysteine is measured in micromoles. Experts consider 9 to 10 micromoles per liter (mol/L) to be normal. Studies suggest that 15 mol/L or higher indicates an increased risk for heart disease. People with high levels of homocysteine may have as much as four times the risk of heart disease as those with normal levels, contributing to the position of many medical experts that high homocysteine may be a marker for increased risk of heart disease.

PART III

CREATING A HEALTHY
LIFESTYLE

CHAPTER 7

Where to Start

You've learned about cholesterol. You've learned about the risk factors. Now it's time to learn what it means to create a healthy overall standard of living. You may not realize how easy it is, with our modern way of life, to fall into an unhealthy existence. Regardless of how difficult the challenge is, though, the rewards of healthy living are worth the commitment and effort. This and the following chapters will provide more specific, practical information on what to eat, how to exercise, and other strategies that will enhance your wellness.

30. Recognize the Downside of Modern Life

One of the greatest ironies of modern living is that it is actually much easier to survive in a manner that contributes to poor health and chronic disease than it is to live a life of vibrant, vital health. The reasons for this are many and complex.

Poor Eating Habits

The foods that are the easiest to obtain and the most plentiful are high-fat, high-sugar, calorie-rich, highly refined processed foods. These foods are often nutrient poor, yet cheap and effortless to find. It takes more time and dedication to find and prepare natural, whole foods.

What you eat has a powerful influence over whether you create a healthy blood lipid profile that includes low LDL cholesterol, high HDL cholesterol, and low triglyceride levels. Research supports that eating a primarily plant-based diet that consists of a large proportion of minimally processed (or whole) grains, vegetables, and fruits is essential to support optimal health.

Lack of Exercise and Excess Weight

Technology has made our lives so easy that it takes perseverance to find opportunities to move. This is not good. To create optimum health, the human body needs to be physically active.

All of this technology means that something we used to take for granted, such as walking around each day to complete our tasks or even to have fun and play, is no longer an essential part of our lives. Instead, we need to plan for movement. We need to brainstorm strategies to stay active. All of this inactivity, combined with easy-to-grab calorie-rich foods, has contributed to weight gain.

Exposure to Toxins

Another aspect of modern living that makes it difficult to support health is that we are exposed to environmental toxins, including numerous carcinogens. Cigarette smoke, air pollution, and other harmful chemicals in our air, water, and food supply undermine our well-being.

Mental Stress

Technology continues to drive the pace of work and living to faster and faster speeds. The cost of living, the pressure of competition for material wealth, and the challenge of balancing family, professional, and community ties all contribute to increasing daily pressures. Finding time to relax, unwind, and savor simple pleasures becomes a rare treat.

In addition to the specific stress-related disorders that this daily pressure causes, stress makes it all the more challenging to actively pursue healthy eating and activity habits. At the end of a long, hard day, it's much easier to grab a fast snack and sit on the couch than to spend time meal-planning, strategizing on how to be more active, and creating time to relax in refreshing and restorative ways.

31. Get Ready for Change

In the field of behavioral medicine, researchers are examining how to support the process of change toward more positive habits. They have realized that changing behaviors is a very difficult task, and they have sought to understand how to improve the process to maximize people's odds of success.

A leading behavioral scientist, James Prochaska, PhD, along with Carlo DiClemente, PhD, developed a psychological model for behavioral change that divides the course of action into five stages of readiness:

- **Precontemplation:** If you are reading this book, you have already progressed beyond this stage. A person in the precontemplation stage is not making and does not intend to make any behavioral changes. A person at this stage is not motivated and does not have the tools and information necessary to make a positive change.
- **Contemplation:** In the contemplation stage, a person knows that it is better to live a healthier lifestyle. Although the person is thinking about it, he or she has not yet taken any action toward making this change a reality. During this stage, a person is engaged in information-gathering and weighing the pros and cons of taking any action.
- **Preparation:** People who are in the preparation stage have already started taking small steps toward acquiring new, healthy habits. For example, if a person wants to be more active, she has gone out and bought a new pair of walking shoes. Or, if a person wants to eat more healthfully, he has purchased a book such as this one, complete with heart-healthy recipes and tips for incorporating better snacking habits.
- **Action:** In the action stage, things start to get exciting. This is the first six-month period of starting up a new exercise program, following a new eating pattern, or integrating new methods of relaxation into your day. Studies show that it typically takes two months to develop a new

habit, and that as many as 50 percent of people who start a new program drop out within the first six months.

- **Maintenance:** The ideal conclusion to a concentrated effort in making a behavioral change is to reach the maintenance phase. In the example of incorporating regular activity, a person gets to the maintenance phase when she has been exercising regularly for at least six months. The odds of giving up this new habit after that length of time are low. The behavior becomes self-motivating because it is easy to feel the benefits and rewards of the healthy activity.

32. Believe in Yourself

Another important concept that researchers have determined is fundamental to successful change is how much you believe in your own ability to achieve it. Self-confidence is important. The more you believe that you can be successful, the more likely you will be successful. In contrast, if you see yourself as a person who simply can't eat nutritious foods or who can't possibly find time to move around more during the day, then it will be true for you. Your perception of yourself is powerful.

Furthermore, the power of your belief in yourself is behavior-specific. For example, you may be very confident that you can walk at least thirty minutes a day on most days of the week. At the same time, you may be very unsure of the fact that you can eat more vegetables and less candy every day. You need to build your confidence in each particular area that you want to succeed. Also, you need to believe that you can achieve the goals that you set for yourself.

33. Identify Your Priorities

Take a few moments to write down the top five things that are important to you. Examples of items you may want to include might be your family, health, community, profession, a hobby, political causes, or volunteer work. Then, on the same piece of paper, list the top five activities that take up most of your time in an average day. Note the percentage of your waking time that they require.

Take a moment to compare how you spend your time each day with what you consider most important in your life. Do you have a good match? Or have you realized that you are neglecting some things that are very important to you? Once you increase your awareness of the way you are spending your time versus the way you want to spend your time, you can start making a difference.

For example, if you realize that you are spending three hours each day watching television and no time walking or participating in any other type of moderate physical activity, you can see that there is some time in your day that you can carve out to use for exercising. If you really can't give up your television time, then consider ways to do some exercises as you watch your favorite programs. Then, try to do this at least four days a week.

34. Enjoy the Fruits of Your Labor

Remember to reward yourself for your good behavior. For example, promise yourself that if you stick to your new eating plan or exercise schedule for four consecutive weeks, you will reward yourself with a nice massage, or buy yourself some new exercise clothing.

Living in a time when we can strive to optimize our health is truly a privilege. When you move about, be aware of the joy of experiencing the sensation of your muscles in action. As you eat a dish of fresh foods, savor the flavors, colors, aroma, and textures that whole foods add to your dining pleasure. And as you feel stronger, more energetic, and simply more alive, know that it is the direct result of your efforts to create a healthy life. You can do it—just keep believing in yourself and in your worth—because you are worth it.

CHAPTER 8

Changing Your Diet

What you put in your body directly creates your health. Dietary factors are associated with four of the ten leading causes of death in the United States: coronary heart disease, stroke, Type 2 diabetes, and certain cancers. The foods you eat can increase or decrease your risk of heart disease, disability, and death. A diet that contributes to atherosclerosis is a major, modifiable risk factor, which means that you can make a powerful difference simply by choosing good foods.

35. Get to Know Dietary Guidelines

In 2000, the American Heart Association issued dietary guidelines to help people follow eating and lifestyle habits to reduce the risk of cardiovascular disease (CVD). In the 2000 guidelines, the American Heart Association strongly endorses "consumption of a diet that contains a variety of foods from all the food categories and emphasizes fruits and vegetables; fat-free and low-fat dairy products; cereal and grain products; legumes and nuts; and fish, poultry, and lean meats." Researchers agree that food-based guidelines are more practical and easier to understand than those that focus on counting calories, fat, or cholesterol.

The American Heart Association guidelines recommend the following foods:

- Five servings of fruits and vegetables a day
- Six servings of grains a day
- Two servings of fatty fish per week
- Include fat-free and low-fat dairy products
- Include legumes (beans)
- Include poultry
- Include lean meats

These guidelines are meant to emphasize the importance of choosing an overall balanced diet with foods from all major food groups, especially fruits, vegetables, and grains. In addition to including the recommended number of servings of the first three types of foods, include balanced amounts of the other foods listed in your meal choices.

The above guidelines are appropriate for everyone age two years and older. Laying the foundation for healthy eating patterns in children is critically important in helping them build healthy habits and in preventing the development of diseases later in life.

36. Choose Good Fat over Bad Fat

When scientists first began investigating the causes of heart disease, fats were identified as an enemy. However, as it turns out, a diet that is higher in fat is actually the primary eating pattern of some of the people with the lowest rates of heart disease. The difference is that the fats include heart-protective vegetable fats. The recognition of the benefits of this style of eating, known as the "Mediterranean diet," represents a landmark change in the thinking about dietary effects on blood lipids. Researchers today support the concept that a primarily plant-based diet, including vegetable oils and fatty fish, is optimal for supporting health.

The Mediterranean Diet

Researchers became intrigued by the diet of southern Europeans when they realized that people from this area enjoyed a very low incidence of heart disease and tended to live longer than North Americans and northern Europeans. The Mediterranean diet is characterized by a high intake of fruits and vegetables, nuts and cereals, and olive oil. In addition, fish and dairy products and wine with meals are regular features. In contrast, the amount of meat and poultry consumed is minimal.

Studies have shown that people placed on a Mediterranean diet can lower their chances of having another heart attack by as much as 67 percent. In another study published in the *New England Journal of Medicine* in 2003, investigators evaluated 22,000 Greek adults over approximately four years and rated the degree to which the participants followed a Mediterranean diet. Scientists found that people who followed the Mediterranean diet closely were 33 percent less likely to die from heart disease and 24 percent less likely to die from cancer when compared to those who did not adhere to a Mediterranean diet.

The Dietary Approaches to Stop Hypertension (DASH) Diet

The DASH study is another significant investigation that supports the value of a diet emphasizing plant-based foods as a way of reducing the risks of high blood pressure. Researchers divided study participants into three groups: a control group; a group that ate a lot of fruits and vegetables; and a combination diet group that ate a lot of fruits and vegetables along with low-fat dairy products.

Investigators found that reductions in blood pressure among the combination diet group were as strong as any single medication. While participants in the fruit and veggie group did experience modest blood pressure reductions, it was not nearly as significant as those who also got calcium and other minerals from the dairy products. Members of the combination diet group also reduced their LDL cholesterol levels 9 percent more than people in the control group. In other words, the risk of heart disease could be reduced through dietary factors alone.

37. Beware of Animal-Based and Processed Foods

To achieve healthy cholesterol levels, the first course of action is to avoid foods with components that elevate LDL cholesterol. This priority comes from the evidence that high total cholesterol and high LDL cholesterol levels increase the risk for heart disease and stroke and that lowering LDL cholesterol levels reduces these risks.

Saturated Fatty Acids

There is a direct relationship between the increased intake of saturated fatty acids, often called saturated fats, and an increase in LDL cholesterol levels. Saturated fatty acids are found in animal-based foods such as meats and dairy products. Steaks and chops, hamburger, sausage, processed meats such as lunchmeat, hot dogs, or salami, and fatty cuts of meat are all common sources of saturated fats, as is the skin on poultry. Dairy products that are rich in saturated fat include cheese, butter, whole milk, 2 percent milk, ice cream, cream, and whole-milk yogurt. Plant-based foods do not contain any saturated fat.

For those who do not have heart disease or high levels of LDL cholesterol, the American Heart Association recommends that saturated fat intake represent less than 10 percent of total calories per day. For those who know they have CVD or who have high LDL cholesterol, the recommendation for daily consumption of saturated fat is much lower, less than 7 percent of total calories.

Trans-Unsaturated Fatty Acids

Trans-unsaturated fatty acids, often referred to as trans fats, are more harmful to your health than saturated fats. As with saturated fats, there is a direct relationship between an increased intake of trans fats and an increase in LDL cholesterol levels. Additionally, a direct relationship exists between increased consumption of trans fats and a reduction in HDL levels.

Trans fats are primarily found in commercially processed foods such as pies, doughnuts, cookies, chips, candy, pastries, shortening, and fried fast foods. Food manufacturers create trans fats through a process called hydrogenation that converts otherwise liquid oils into a more solid substance. This hydrogenation is useful to food manufacturers because it increases the shelf life of foods, adds form to otherwise liquid substances, and adds flavor.

According to a report by the Institute of Medicine, a nonprofit organization chartered by the National Academy of Sciences, there is a direct relationship between the consumption of trans fatty acids and an increase in total cholesterol and LDL levels. This means that consuming trans fatty acids increases the risk of coronary heart disease and should therefore be avoided.

Cholesterol from Animal-Based Foods

Just as the cells in the human body contain cholesterol, so do the cells of all other animals. Plants and plant-based foods, however, contain no cholesterol. A good rule of thumb to remember is that many foods that are high in saturated fats are also high in cholesterol. Cholesterol-rich foods include organ meats (such as liver), certain shellfish, poultry, dairy products, and eggs. A recent study, however, showed that consumption of one egg per day by a person who does not have known CVD or elevated lipid levels did not contribute to elevated blood cholesterol levels.

Eating foods high in cholesterol can increase LDL cholesterol levels, but not nearly as much as eating foods high in saturated fats and trans fats can. In other words, you will improve your cholesterol levels more by cutting down on foods high in saturated and trans fats than by reducing consumption of foods that contain cholesterol.

38. Eat Your Fruits and Veggies

Studies show that dietary patterns that include a high consumption of fruits and vegetables are associated with lower risks of developing heart disease, stroke, and hypertension. Unlike many high-fat and high-sugar processed foods, fresh fruits and vegetables are nutrient-dense and low in calories. Fruits and vegetables are also high in water content. This helps to maintain adequate hydration levels and contributes to feelings of fullness. This type of eating pattern will provide you with plenty of healthy fiber, essential nutrients, and beneficial phytochemicals and antioxidants.

Phytochemicals are chemicals that give plants color and assist in keeping the plants healthy. In the same way that phytochemicals fight disease, oxidation, and inflammation in plants, they are also beneficial for human health. Various phytochemicals support heart health through different protective actions. Antioxidants such as certain vitamins, carotenoids, and flavonoids prevent oxidation and decrease the likelihood of oxidized LDL cholesterol sticking to arterial walls. Vitamins C and E are rich sources of antioxidants.

Vegetables and fruits are also a rich source of vitamin B complex. Folate in particular is essential to health, as it helps to prevent high levels of harmful homocysteine from circulating in the bloodstream and damaging arterial walls. Eating foods rich in folate prevents high levels of homocysteine. While it is not yet proven by research that treating elevated homocysteine levels reduces the risk of heart disease, we do know that elevated levels are a marker for increased heart disease risk. Foods rich in folate include beans, asparagus, fresh leafy greens, and oranges.

Other minerals play a valuable role in regulating blood pressure and in keeping blood vessels healthy. Minerals such as calcium, magnesium, and potassium can help keep blood vessels relaxed and blood pressure under control. Food sources of calcium, magnesium, and potassium include artichokes, cantaloupes, broccoli, bananas, cauliflower, bell peppers, and many others.

39. Discover Whole Grains

Whole grains provide fiber, vitamins, complex carbohydrates, and minerals. Studies show that people who consume more whole grains have a lower risk of heart disease. A whole grain still contains the outer shell, or bran, of the grain and the germ, which would turn into a seedling. Whole grains are superior to processed grains because many nutrients are lost during refining.

When you purchase grain products, look for the terms "whole," "whole wheat," or "whole grain" before the name of the grain in the list of ingredients to ensure that you are getting the best nutritional value for your money. If you must eat processed grains, be sure to choose those that have been enriched with vitamins, particularly with B vitamins, to replace those lost during refining.

---

did you know . . . ?

Since grains are rich in fiber and low in fat, they also contribute to a healthy, lower calorie diet. Therefore, when you eat the recommended amounts of grains, you feel full without having consumed excess calories. This contrasts greatly to the typical highly processed and refined foods that are quickly digested, are high in calories, and do not provide the same feelings of satiety.

Diets high in simple carbohydrates, such as white flours and pasta, can lead to elevated triglyceride levels and reduced levels of HDL (good) cholesterol. This increases risks to cardiovascular health and explains why dietary recommendations no longer advise severely limited fat intake and high carbohydrate consumption. Importantly, this adverse effect does not occur when the carbohydrates in the diet come from complex carbohydrate sources such as whole grains. Therefore, you should eat whole grains for optimal health and avoid highly refined grains as much as possible.

40. Add More Nutrients to Your Diet

When you choose plant-based and whole foods, there are several important nutrients that become part of your diet. These include soluble fiber found in plant-based foods and omega-3 fatty acids found in fish.

Soluble Fiber

Increasing soluble fiber by only 5 to 10 grams per day is shown to reduce LDL cholesterol by as much as 5 percent. Even more significant reductions in cholesterol level can be achieved by increasing the daily intake to 10 to 25 grams per day. Whole wheat, whole oats, barley, rye, oat bran, rice bran, corn bran, and psyllium seeds all contain soluble fiber. Certain fruits, such as apples, prunes, pears, and oranges, also contain soluble fiber.

The reason that soluble fiber helps to lower LDL cholesterol is that, in the intestines, soluble fiber binds with cholesterol, making it unable to be absorbed by the body. The cholesterol is then excreted in your bowel movement, forcing the liver to dip into its cholesterol reserves to manufacture more bile acids for digestion, resulting in an overall reduction in cholesterol in the body.

did you know . . . ?

Eating soluble-fiber-rich foods such as oat products, psyllium seeds, pectin (in apples and other fruit), and guar gum reduces LDL cholesterol, particularly in people with high cholesterol. Studies show that for about each gram of soluble fiber eaten daily, LDL cholesterol drops an average of 2.2 mg/dL. Furthermore, high-fiber diets do not reduce HDL cholesterol or elevate triglycerides.

Omega-3 Polyunsaturated Fatty Acids

Studies show that consumption of foods rich in omega-3 fatty acids offers multiple benefits for heart health. Positive effects include reducing triglyceride levels, reducing risk of sudden cardiac death, reducing blood-clotting tendencies, improving blood vessel dilation, and lowering the risk of arrhythmia (irregular heartbeat). Fish is also a good source of protein that does not contain harmful saturated animal fats. Deep-water fish such as salmon, tuna, herring, and mackerel are particularly good dietary sources of omega-3 fatty acids. Other plant-based sources include flaxseed and flaxseed oil, canola oil, soybean oil, and nuts.

Soy Protein

A review article of thirty-one studies on soy and cholesterol published in the *New England Journal of Medicine* concluded, "Eating soy in place of animal protein lowers high cholesterol, which may reduce one's risk of heart disease by 10 to 30 percent." Based on these studies, the FDA has approved a health claim on food labels that consuming 25 grams of soy protein daily reduces the risk of heart disease, primarily due to its effect on blood cholesterol.

The reason that dietary soy protein is beneficial to health may be that soy is rich in phytoestrogen isoflavones, or plant estrogens, that can have a heart-protective effect similar to human estrogen.

Plant Stanols and Sterols

Plant stanols and sterols are components that are isolated from the oil of soybeans and of tall pine trees. They are phytochemicals, or chemicals from plants. These are then added as a supplement to certain foods.

Cholesterol is an animal sterol that serves as an integral part of the structure of cell membranes in animals; plant sterols serve the same role in the cell membranes of plants. Because of their structural similarity to cholesterol, plant sterols and stanols will bind with cholesterol during the digestive process. But their subtle differences from cholesterol keep plant sterols from being easily absorbed through the human intestine. Therefore, if a plant sterol binds with cholesterol, it effectively blocks the absorption of that cholesterol through the intestine and promotes its excretion from the body, thus lowering cholesterol levels that circulate in the bloodstream.

Monounsaturated Vegetable Fats

Research shows that a diet that includes monounsaturated fats reduces total cholesterol and LDL cholesterol levels and has no effect on good cholesterol levels. Nor does consuming foods rich in monounsaturated fats raise triglycerides. This heart-protective effect of monounsaturated fats is believed to partly explain why people who follow a Mediterranean diet that is rich in olive oil live long and healthy lives. Monounsaturated fats are liquid at room temperature and include fats from vegetables and nuts. Foods that are rich in monounsaturated fats include nuts, avocados, and plant oils such as olive, canola, and peanut.

CHAPTER 9

Strategies for Healthy Eating

Knowing what foods are good for you is only half the story; figuring out how to eat them regularly is the challenging part. Changing your routine is never easy, but you can do it if you keep taking small steady steps. The tips in this chapter will help you to move toward a healthier pattern of eating. Once you start feeling the benefits of enjoying fresher and more wholesome foods, your new habits will be self-reinforcing.

41. Prioritize Plant-Based Foods

The connection between food and your blood cholesterol levels is direct and powerful. Overconsumption of saturated fats, trans fats, and cholesterol-rich foods leads to overproduction of LDL cholesterol in the liver and to the release of excess amounts of triglycerides into the bloodstream. Saturated fats and cholesterol are only present in animal foods. Trans fats are only present in processed, commercial foods.

When you alter your eating habits to include more plant-based foods and fewer animal-based and processed foods, you take a powerful step toward improving the health of your bloodstream. Studies have shown that nutritional factors alone can reduce total blood cholesterol by as much as 30 percent in individuals with high levels of cholesterol. This change is almost as powerful as the best prescription medications. The significant difference is that improvements in nutrition do not have the same risk of adverse side effects as taking a long-term prescription drug. Furthermore, the nutritional remedy is much more affordable.

Numerous nutritional studies demonstrate that plant-based foods enhance our health, particularly cardiovascular health. Humans cannot exist without plant foods. While it is possible to live healthfully over a lifetime without any consumption of meat, it is not possible to survive without eating plant-based foods.

42. Move Away from Meats and Animal Fats

You can enjoy meat as part of a heart-healthy diet; you just need to use it carefully. Ways to do this include creating dishes from lean cuts of meats and enjoying meats as more of a side dish than a main course. Also, purchase meats that have been fed grass diets, also called "free range," rather than animal fats and animal byproducts.

just the facts

Cows are naturally grass-eating animals. Meat from grass-fed cattle has about one-half to one-third the fat as meat from grain-fed cattle. Grass-fed beef is lower in calories, and higher in vitamin E, omega-3 fatty acids, and conjugated linoleic acid, another health-enhancing fatty acid. Ask your grocer for grass-fed or free-range beef.

Reduce Saturated Fat in Meats

When you prepare meats, try to do so in a manner that reduces rather than increases the amount of fat. For example, baste with wines or marinades and season with herbs; grill or broil meats instead of frying or breading; sauté or brown meats in pans sprayed with vegetable oils. If you are adding meat to other dishes, such as spaghetti, brown it first and pour off the fat before you add it to the sauce. Here are some more meat preparation tips:

- Trim excess fat from meats.
- Remove skin from poultry.
- Broil, grill, roast, or bake meats on racks that allow fats to drain off.
- Avoid organ meats completely, such as livers, brains, sweetbreads, and kidneys.

- Skim fats from tops of stews or casseroles.
- Also avoid (completely, if you can) processed meats, such as lunch-meat, salami, bologna, pepperoni, or sausage.

Lower Saturated Fats in Dairy Products

Eating full-fat dairy products increases the levels of saturated fat in your diet, which directly increases your levels of LDL or bad cholesterol. You can still enjoy dairy foods. Simply choose nonfat versions to promote health, and choose products from dairy cows that have been fed grass diets.

Cheese, in particular, is a very high-fat food. While a rare treat of a creamy cheese is not going to harm your overall health, indulging in them regularly will definitely increase your risk of heart disease. Here are some practical tips on lowering the amount of saturated dairy fat in your diet:

- Choose nonfat, ½ percent, or 1 percent milk, preferably from grass-fed cows.
- Select nonfat or low-fat yogurt, sour cream, and cottage and cream cheese.
- Use lower fat cheeses for cooking, such as part-skim mozzarella, ricotta, or Parmesan.
- Enjoy rich, creamy, and hard cheeses only on special occasions.
- Limit the use of butter. Use the canola-based butter instead.

Check that dairy products come from cows fed grasses and grains rather than meat byproducts. Look for other sources of calcium in your diet. Vegetables such as broccoli, chard, greens, and artichokes are all great sources of dietary calcium, as well as calcium-fortified orange juice and some whole-grain cereals.

Avoid Trans Fats

Trans fats increase your LDL cholesterol and decrease your HDL cholesterol levels. They are found naturally in some dairy and meat products, but most trans fats in the food supply have been created artificially through a process called hydrogenation, which converts a liquid fat to a solid.

Trans fats are abundant in processed foods such as cereals, chips, crackers, stick margarine, shortening, lard, and fried fast foods. Remember that trans fats can be manufactured from vegetable oils, so simply because a food manufacturer indicates that something is prepared with vegetable oil does not mean that it is trans fat free.

Avoid using foods with ingredients such as hydrogenated or partially hydrogenated oils. If you must buy a product with such an ingredient, ensure that the hydrogenated ingredient appears at the end of the ingredient list, indicating that it is present in very low quantities.

43. Consider These Quick Ways to Eat More Fruits and Vegetables

Try to incorporate fruits or vegetables at every meal and as snacks. Reduce the amount of meat or chicken in typical combination dishes. For example, in spaghetti, reduce the amount of beef or substitute ground turkey. Then increase the vegetable content in your sauces by adding more mushrooms, green peppers, celery, and carrots.

Here are more tips on how to include more vegetables in your daily diet:

- At breakfast, slice half a banana or toss some berries or raisins on your cereal.
- For a mid-morning snack, try chopped carrots and celery with a glass of vegetable juice.
- At meals, serve larger portions of vegetables, or prepare multiple vegetable dishes, and have meat as a side dish.
- Prepare meats with fruit toppings or marinades instead of butter.
- Enjoy fruit-based desserts such as poached pears, baked apples, or fresh fruit sorbets.
- Buy packaged, prewashed, and sliced veggies to pack as snacks or to eat at lunch.
- Eat fresh whole fruits that are in season as snacks.
- Add vegetables such as peas into rice or pasta dishes.
- Incorporate multiple vegetables into salads in addition to lettuce.
- Enjoy a smoothie made with fruits or vegetables as a snack.

44. Enjoy Whole-Grain Foods

Whole-grain foods are minimally processed and therefore rich in vitamins, minerals, and fiber. Grains include whole wheat, brown rice, barley, rye, oatmeal, and corn. Whole grains provide complex carbohydrates that are essential for energy, and vitamins A and E, magnesium, calcium, and other important nutrients. These fiber-rich foods contain both soluble and insoluble fiber, but mostly contain insoluble fiber, which aids digestion, keeps your colon healthy, and makes you feel full, helping with weight management. Processed grains, in contrast, are simple carbohydrates and have lost many of the nutrients and the fiber.

Oatmeal that contains oat bran is a rich source of soluble fiber that can help to lower cholesterol levels. Food manufacturers often remove the oat bran in the instant-cook varieties. Be sure to purchase whole oats or oat bran to obtain the cholesterol-lowering results.

Ideally, you should eat six servings of grains per day. Here are some tips to add more whole grains into your daily diet:

- Include a grain-based food at every meal.
- Try whole-grain rolls, breadsticks, and muffins for snacks.
- Purchase whole-grain crackers for meals or snacks.
- Enjoy rice cakes or popcorn that do not include trans fats for snacks.
- Prepare desserts with fruits and whole grains, such as apple crisp.
- Sprinkle wheat germ into your cereals or smoothies.
- Use whole-grain tortillas or pita breads to make healthy chips for dips or salsas.

45. Learn to Read Food Labels

The FDA regulates food labels. Labels must include not only a list of nutrients but also a list of ingredients. These are both sources of valuable information. In the nutrient list, the important items to check include the total fats and the breakdown of the types of fats included, as well as the total carbohydrates and breakdown of fiber and sugar.

In the total fat section, check to see how much saturated fat and total fat are listed. Remember, "bad" fats that you should limit or avoid include saturated fat, trans fat, and—to a limited extent—cholesterol. "Good" fats that you should include are monounsaturated and polyunsaturated fats.

In the carbohydrate section of the label, check how much dietary fiber and sugar is in the product. Select foods that are higher in dietary fiber and as low as possible in sugar. When making a buying decision, compare products to find those that contain good fats instead of bad fats and that are high in fiber and whole grains.

The ingredient list also provides a wealth of valuable information. Ingredients are listed in order of magnitude, with the items used in larger amounts listed first and smallest amounts at the end. Try to choose foods that feature the fat and oil ingredients toward the end of the list.

Choose products that list the specific type of vegetable oil—soybean oil, for example—rather than labels that use a generic "vegetable oil" listing. Often when manufacturers use the term "vegetable oil," the product includes tropical oils such as palm or coconut that contain saturated fats, rather than the healthier monounsaturated and polyunsaturated fats. To avoid trans fats, stay away from products that list hydrogenated or partially hydrogenated vegetable oils.

When it comes to grain products, choose products with the words "whole," "whole wheat," or "whole grain" in front of the grain ingredient, as well as terms like "bran" or "germ."

46. Plan Your Meals

Maintaining healthy nutrition does require some planning. However, with a minimal amount of organization, you can keep health-enhancing foods in your refrigerator and cupboards. Now let's look at how you can use these tips to plan healthy meals.

Breakfast

Breakfast is the most important meal of the day. It's also a wonderful opportunity to eat fiber-rich foods. Plan to include a combination of fiber-rich and protein-rich foods, along with either a fruit or vegetable serving. Great sources of fiber for breakfast include hot or cold cereals and breads. Breakfast protein can come from nonfat or low-fat dairy products such as milk or soy-milk. You can add fruits or vegetables either by drinking one glass of juice or by mixing fruit with your cereal dish.

Another excellent breakfast option is a smoothie. These are easy to make in a blender, with either milk or soymilk, some fruits, and wheat germ or ground flaxseed.

Lunch

Lunch is another opportunity for a rich source of fiber and more fruits and vegetables. Try sandwiches on hearty whole-grain breads with fresh toma-toes, lettuce, and sprouts. For vegetable sources of protein, use bean dips such as hummus on the sandwich. Peanut butter is also a good sandwich filling, or you might try avocados.

If packing a lunch, include a vegetable and some fruit. For example, take some prewashed, prepackaged baby carrots or celery sticks. Or slice up a bell pepper into sticks. Easily portable fruits include apples, bananas, oranges, nectarines, grapes, and pears.

Salads are a great lunch that can be made more filling by adding beans, hard-boiled eggs, or starches such as whole-grain pastas. You can also add cubes of tofu or tempeh to your salads. Tofu can also be added to steamed vegetables, soup, and sauces. Soups are a fantastic source of multiple vegetables and beans.

Dinner

For dinner, try to shift the emphasis to a vegetable- and grain-based main course with any meat dishes on the side. Or, in meals that call for sauces, use a combination of vegetables and meats to reduce the total amount of meat that you consume. For example, cut the amount of meat in stew in half and instead add in extra carrots, celery, and mushrooms. You can try chili with beans and no meat, or use ground turkey instead of beef and add more vegetables instead of meats. Try enjoying stir-fried vegetable dishes with only a small amount of skinless chicken, or simply use tofu instead of any meat product.

Keep in mind that when you eat beans, peas, or lentils together with a dairy product or with grains such as bread or rice, you can obtain the same amount of protein from your meal as if you had consumed a meat dish.

PART IV

HEART-HEALTHY RECIPES

CHAPTER 10

Soup, Appetizer, and Side Dish Recipes

The heart-healthy recipes in this and the following chapters will help you plan tasty, enjoyable, and nutritious meals for your entire family. These recipes, from the National Heart, Lung, and Blood Institute, were developed under the direction of leading medical and nutritional scientists during government-sponsored research and education projects devoted to keeping Americans healthy.

47. Corn Chowder

Makes 4 servings (Serving size: 1 cup)

Here's a creamy chowder without the cream—or fat.

1 tablespoon vegetable oil
2 tablespoons celery, finely diced
2 tablespoons onion, finely diced
2 tablespoons green pepper, finely diced
1 package (10 ounce) frozen whole-kernel corn
1 cup raw potatoes, peeled, diced in ½-inch pieces
1 cup water
¼ teaspoon salt
Black pepper to taste
¼ teaspoon paprika
2 cups low-fat or skim milk
2 tablespoons flour
2 tablespoons fresh parsley, chopped

1. Heat oil in medium saucepan. Add celery, onion, and green pepper, and sauté for 2 minutes.
2. Add corn, potatoes, water, salt, pepper, and paprika. Bring to boil, then reduce heat to medium. Cook covered for about 10 minutes or until potatoes are tender.
3. Place ½ cup of milk in jar with tight-fitting lid. Add flour and shake vigorously.
4. Gradually add milk-flour mixture to cooked vegetables. Then add remaining milk.
5. Cook, stirring constantly, until mixture comes to boil and thickens.
6. Serve garnished with chopped fresh parsley.

EACH SERVING PROVIDES:			
Calories: 186	Cholesterol: 5 mg	Protein: 7 g
Total fat: 5 g	Sodium: 205 mg	Carbohydrates: 31 g
Saturated fat: 1 g	Total fiber: 4 g	Potassium: 455 mg

48. Homemade Turkey Soup

Makes 6 servings (about 4 quarts of soup)
(Serving size: 1 cup)

*This popular soup uses a "quick cooldown" method
that lets you skim the fat right off the top.*

6 pounds turkey breast with bones
  (with at least 2 cups meat)
2 medium onions
3 stalks celery
1 teaspoon dried thyme
½ teaspoon dried rosemary
½ teaspoon dried sage
1 teaspoon dried basil
½ teaspoon dried marjoram
½ teaspoon dried tarragon
½ teaspoon salt
Black pepper, to taste
½ pound Italian pastina or pasta

1. Place turkey breast in large 6-quart pot. Cover with water until at least three-quarters full.
2. Peel onions, cut into large pieces, and add to pot. Wash celery stalks, slice, and add to pot.
3. Simmer covered for about 2½ hours.
4. Remove carcass from pot. Divide soup into smaller, shallower containers for quick cooling in refrigerator.
5. After cooling, skim off fat.
6. While soup cools, remove remaining meat from turkey carcass. Cut into pieces.
7. Add turkey meat to skimmed soup, along with herbs and spices.
8. Bring to boil and add pastina. Continue cooking on low boil for about 20 minutes, until pastina is done. Serve at once or refrigerate for later reheating.

EACH SERVING PROVIDES:			
	Calories: 201	Cholesterol: 101 mg	Protein: 33 g
	Total fat: 2 g	Sodium: 141 mg	Carbohydrates: 11 g
	Saturated fat: 1 g	Total fiber: 1 g	Potassium: 344 mg

49. Pupusas Revueltas

Makes 12 servings (Serving size: 2 pupusas)

*Ground chicken and low-fat cheese help keep
down the fat and calories in this tasty dish.*

1 pound chicken breast, ground
1 tablespoon vegetable oil
½ small onion, finely diced
1 clove garlic, minced
1 medium green pepper, seeded,
   minced
1 small tomato, finely chopped
5 cups instant corn flour (masa harina)
6 cups water
½ pound low-fat mozzarella cheese,
   grated

1. In nonstick skillet, sauté chicken in oil over low heat until it turns white. Stir chicken to keep it from sticking.
2. Add onion, garlic, green pepper, and tomato. Cook chicken mixture through. Remove skillet from heat and refrigerate.
3. Place flour in large mixing bowl and add water to make stiff, tortilla-like dough.
4. When chicken mixture has cooled, mix in cheese.
5. Divide dough into 24 portions. Shape dough into balls and flatten each into ½-inch thick circle. Put spoonful of chicken mixture in middle of each circle of dough and bring edges to center. Flatten ball of dough again until it is ½-inch thick.
6. In very hot iron skillet, cook pupusas on each side until golden brown.
7. Serve hot.

EACH SERVING PROVIDES:			
Calories: 290	Cholesterol: 33 mg	Protein: 14 g
Total fat: 7 g	Sodium: 223 mg	Carbohydrates: 38 g
Saturated fat: 3 g	Total fiber: 5 g	Potassium: 272 mg

50. Italian Vegetable Bake

Makes 18 servings (Serving size: ½ cup)

Try this colorful, low-sodium baked dish, prepared without added fat.

1 can (28 ounces) tomatoes, whole
1 medium onion, sliced
½ pound fresh green beans, sliced
½ pound fresh okra, cut into ½-inch pieces (or ½ of 10-ounce package frozen, cut)
¾ cup green pepper, finely chopped
2 tablespoons lemon juice
1 tablespoon fresh basil, chopped, or 1 teaspoon dried basil, crushed
1½ teaspoons fresh oregano leaves, chopped (or ½ teaspoon dried oregano, crushed)
3 medium (7-inch-long) zucchini, cut into 1-inch cubes
1 medium eggplant, pared, cut into 1-inch cubes
2 tablespoons Parmesan cheese, grated

1. Drain and coarsely chop tomatoes. Save liquid. Mix together tomatoes, reserved liquid, onion, green beans, okra, green pepper, lemon juice, and herbs. Cover and bake at 325°F for 15 minutes.
2. Mix in zucchini and eggplant. Continue baking, covered, 60 to 70 minutes more or until vegetables are tender. Stir occasionally.
3. Just before serving, sprinkle top with Parmesan cheese.

EACH SERVING PROVIDES:			
Calories: 27	Cholesterol: 1 mg	Protein: 2 g
Total fat: less than 1 g	Sodium: 86 mg	Carbohydrates: 5 g
Saturated fat: less than 1 g	Total fiber: 2 g	Potassium: 244 mg

51. Wonderful Stuffed Potatoes

Makes 8 servings (Serving size: ½ potato)

These stuffed potatoes make a delicious side dish and you won't miss the sour cream and bacon of the traditional (and far less healthy) version.

4 medium baking potatoes
¾ cup low-fat (1%) cottage cheese
¼ cup low-fat (1%) milk
2 tablespoons soft margarine
1 teaspoon dill weed
¾ teaspoon herb seasoning
4–6 drops hot pepper sauce
2 teaspoons Parmesan cheese, grated

1. Prick potatoes with fork. Bake at 425°F for 60 minutes or until fork is easily inserted.
2. Cut potatoes in half lengthwise. Carefully scoop out potato, leaving about ½ inch of pulp inside shell. Mash pulp in large bowl.
3. By hand, mix in remaining ingredients, except Parmesan cheese. Spoon mixture into potato shells.
4. Sprinkle each top with ¼ teaspoon Parmesan cheese.
5. Place on baking sheet and return to oven. Bake for 15 to 20 minutes or until tops are golden brown.

EACH SERVING PROVIDES:		
Calories: 113	Cholesterol: 1 mg	Protein: 5 g
Total fat: 3 g	Sodium: 151 mg	Carbohydrates: 17 g
Saturated fat: 1 g	Total fiber: 2 g	Potassium: 293 mg

CHAPTER 11

Meat and Poultry Main Dish Recipes

The following are some more great recipes that have been specifically designed and tested to promote health. This collection includes a variety of ethnic dishes to please every taste. Even children love these recipes. In addition, each recipe includes a nutrient breakdown so you know exactly what you're eating. Remember, heart-healthy cooking does not mean a sacrifice of flavor or pleasure.

52. Bavarian Beef

Makes 5 servings (Serving size: 5 ounces)

*This classic German stew is made with lean,
trimmed beef stew meat and cabbage.*

1¼ pounds lean beef stew meat,
   trimmed of fat, cut in 1-inch pieces
1 tablespoon vegetable oil
1 large onion, thinly sliced
1½ cups water
¾ teaspoon caraway seeds
½ teaspoon salt
⅛ teaspoon black pepper
1 bay leaf
¼ cup white vinegar
1 tablespoon sugar
½ small head red cabbage, cut into
   4 wedges
¼ cup gingersnaps, crushed

1. Brown meat in oil in heavy skillet.
   Remove meat and sauté onion in remaining oil until golden. Return meat to skillet.
   Add water, caraway seeds, salt, pepper, and bay leaf. Bring to boil. Reduce heat, cover, and simmer for 1¼ hours.
2. Add vinegar and sugar, and stir. Place cabbage on top of meat. Cover and simmer for an added 45 minutes.
3. Remove meat and cabbage, arrange on platter, and keep warm.
4. Strain drippings from skillet and skim off fat. Add enough water to drippings to yield 1 cup of liquid.
5. Return to skillet with crushed gingersnaps. Cook and stir until thickened and mixture boils. Pour over meat and vegetables, and serve.

EACH SERVING PROVIDES:			
Calories: 218	Cholesterol: 60 mg	Protein: 24 g
Total fat: 7 g	Sodium: 323 mg	Carbohydrates: 14 g
Saturated fat: 2 g	Total fiber: 2 g	Potassium: 509 mg

53. Stir-Fried Beef and Potatoes

Makes 6 servings (Serving size: 1¼ cups)

Vinegar and garlic give this easy-to-fix dish its tasty zip.

1½ pounds sirloin steak
2 teaspoons vegetable oil
1 clove garlic, minced
1 teaspoon vinegar
⅛ teaspoon salt
⅛ teaspoon pepper
2 large onions, sliced
1 large tomato, sliced
3 cups boiled potatoes, diced

1. Trim fat from steak and cut into small, thin pieces.
2. In large skillet, heat oil and sauté garlic until golden.
3. Add steak, vinegar, salt, and pepper. Cook for 6 minutes, stirring beef until brown.
4. Add onion and tomato. Cook until onion is transparent. Serve with boiled potatoes.

EACH SERVING PROVIDES			
Calories: 274	Cholesterol: 56 mg	Protein: 24 g
Total fat: 5 g	Sodium: 96 mg	Carbohydrates: 33 g
Saturated fat: 1 g	Total fiber: 3 g	Potassium: 878 mg

54. Baked Pork Chops

Makes 6 servings (Serving size: 1 chop)

Sink your chops into these pork chops made spicy and moist with a lively blend of herbs. Try with skinless, boneless chicken, turkey, or fish.

6 lean center-cut pork chops, ½-inch
   thick
1 egg white
1 cup evaporated skim milk
¾ cup cornflake crumbs
¼ cup fine dry bread crumbs
4 teaspoons paprika
2 teaspoons oregano
¾ teaspoon chili powder
½ teaspoon garlic powder
½ teaspoon black pepper
⅛ teaspoon cayenne pepper
⅛ teaspoon dry mustard
½ teaspoon salt
Nonstick cooking spray as needed

1. Preheat oven to 375°F.
2. Trim fat from pork chops.
3. Beat egg white with evaporated skim milk. Place chops in milk mixture and let stand for 5 minutes, turning once.
4. Meanwhile, mix cornflake crumbs, bread crumbs, spices, and salt.
5. Use nonstick cooking spray on 13" × 9" baking pan.
6. Remove chops from milk mixture and coat thoroughly with crumb mixture.
7. Place chops in pan and bake at 375°F for 20 minutes.
8. Turn chops and bake for additional 15 minutes or until no pink remains.

EACH SERVING PROVIDES:			
Calories: 216	Cholesterol: 62 mg	Protein: 25 g
Total fat: 8 g	Sodium: 346 mg	Carbohydrates: 10 g
Saturated fat: 3 g	Total fiber: 1 g	Potassium: 414 mg

55. Chicken Gumbo

Makes 8 servings (Serving size: ¾ cup)

Simple but filling—this dish feeds the need.

1 teaspoon vegetable oil
¼ cup flour
3 cups low-sodium chicken broth
1½ pounds chicken breast, skinless, boneless, cut into 1-inch strips
1 cup (½ pound) white potatoes, cubed
1 cup onions, chopped
1 cup (½ pound) carrots, coarsely chopped
½ medium carrot, grated
¼ cup celery, chopped
4 cloves garlic, finely minced
2 scallions, chopped
1 whole bay leaf
½ teaspoon thyme
½ teaspoon black pepper, ground
2 teaspoons hot (or jalapeño) pepper
1 cup (½ pound) okra, sliced into ½-inch pieces

1. Add oil to large pot and heat over medium flame.
2. Stir in flour. Cook, stirring constantly, until flour begins to turn golden brown.
3. Slowly stir in all broth using wire whisk. Cook for 2 minutes. Broth mixture should not be lumpy.
4. Add rest of ingredients except okra. Bring to boil, then reduce heat and let simmer for 20 to 30 minutes.
5. Add okra and let cook for 15 to 20 more minutes.
6. Remove bay leaf and serve hot in bowl or over rice.

EACH SERVING PROVIDES:			
Calories: 165	Cholesterol: 51 mg	Protein: 21 g
Total fat: 4 g	Sodium: 81 mg	Carbohydrates: 11 g
Saturated fat: 1 g	Total fiber: 2 g	Potassium: 349 mg

56. Finger-Licking Curried Chicken

Makes 6 servings (Serving size: ½ breast or 2 small drumsticks)

The name tells all—ginger and curry powder make this dish irresistible.

1½ teaspoons curry powder
1 teaspoon thyme, crushed
1 scallion, chopped
1 tablespoon jalapeño, chopped
1 teaspoon black pepper, ground
8 cloves garlic, crushed
1 tablespoon ginger, grated
1 large onion, chopped
¾ teaspoon salt
8 pieces chicken, skinless (breast and drumstick)
1 tablespoon olive oil
1 cup water
1 medium white potato, diced

1. Mix together curry powder, thyme, scallion, jalapeño, black pepper, garlic, ginger, onion, and salt.
2. Sprinkle seasoning mixture on chicken.
3. Allow rub to sit on chicken for at least 2 hours in refrigerator.
4. Heat oil in skillet over medium flame. Add chicken and sauté.
5. Add water and allow chicken to cook over medium flame for 30 minutes.
6. Add diced potatoes and cook for an additional 30 minutes.
7. Add onions and cook for 15 minutes more or until meat is tender.

EACH SERVING PROVIDES:			
Calories: 213	Cholesterol: 81 mg	Protein: 28 g
Total fat: 6 g	Sodium: 363 mg	Carbohydrates: 10 g
Saturated fat: 2 g	Total fiber: 1 g	Potassium: 384 mg

CHAPTER 12

Fish, Pasta, and Bean Main Dish Recipes

Here are some more delicious recipes to add to your culinary repertoire. You've read about all the benefits of including fish and beans in your diet; this is your chance to put your knowledge into action. This chapter will also help you use pastas in a healthy way. Whole-grain pastas can make a tasty, nutritious addition to your meals.

57. Baked Salmon Dijon

Makes 6 servings
(Serving size: 1 4-ounce piece)

*This salmon entrée is easy to make and
will be enjoyed by the whole family!*

1 cup fat-free sour cream
2 teaspoons dried dill
3 tablespoons scallions, finely chopped
2 tablespoons Dijon mustard
2 tablespoons lemon juice
1½ pounds salmon fillet with skin, cut in center
½ teaspoon garlic powder
½ teaspoon black pepper
Fat-free cooking spray, as needed

1. Whisk sour cream, dill, scallions, mustard, and lemon juice in small bowl to blend.
2. Preheat oven to 400°F. Lightly oil baking sheet with cooking spray.
3. Place salmon, skin side down, on prepared sheet. Sprinkle with garlic powder and pepper, then spread with the sauce.
4. Bake salmon until just opaque in center, about 20 minutes.

EACH SERVING PROVIDES:			
Calories: 196	Cholesterol: 76 mg	Protein: 27 g
Total fat: 7 g	Sodium: 229 mg	Carbohydrates: 5 g
Saturated fat: 2 g	Total fiber: less than 1 g	Potassium: 703 mg

58. Mediterranean Baked Fish

Makes 4 servings (Serving size: 1 4-ounce fillet with sauce)

Taste the Mediterranean in this dish's tomato, onion, and garlic sauce.

2 teaspoons olive oil
1 large onion, sliced
1 can (16 ounces) whole tomatoes, drained (juice reserved), coarsely chopped
½ cup tomato juice (reserved from canned tomatoes)
1 bay leaf
1 clove garlic, minced
1 cup dry white wine
¼ cup lemon juice
¼ cup orange juice
1 tablespoon fresh orange peel, grated
1 teaspoon fennel seeds, crushed
½ teaspoon dried oregano, crushed
½ teaspoon dried thyme, crushed
½ teaspoon dried basil, crushed
Black pepper to taste
1 pound fish fillets (sole, flounder, or sea perch)

1. Heat oil in large nonstick skillet. Add onion and sauté over moderate heat for 5 minutes or until soft.
2. Add all remaining ingredients except fish. Stir well and simmer uncovered for 30 minutes.
3. Arrange fish in 10" × 6" baking dish. Cover with sauce. Bake uncovered at 375°F for about 15 minutes or until fish flakes easily.

EACH SERVING PROVIDES:		
Calories: 178	Cholesterol: 56 mg	Protein: 22 g
Total fat: 4 g	Sodium: 260 mg	Carbohydrates: 12 g
Saturated fat: 1 g	Total fiber: 3 g	Potassium: 678 mg

59. Scallop Kebabs

Makes 4 servings
(Serving size: 1 6-ounce kebab)

*These colorful kebabs use scallops,
which are naturally low in saturated fat.*

3 medium green peppers, cut into
    1½-inch squares
1½ pounds fresh bay scallops
1 pint cherry tomatoes
¼ cup dry white wine
¼ cup vegetable oil
3 tablespoons lemon juice
Dash garlic powder
Black pepper to taste
4 skewers

1. Parboil green peppers for 2 minutes.
2. Alternately thread first three ingredients on skewers.
3. Combine next five ingredients.
4. Brush kebabs with wine/oil/lemon mixture, then place on grill (or under broiler).
5. Grill for 15 minutes, turning and basting frequently.

EACH SERVING PROVIDES:			
	Calories: 224	Cholesterol: 43 mg	Protein: 30 g
	Total fat: 6 g	Sodium: 355 mg	Carbohydrates: 13 g
	Saturated fat: 1 g	Total fiber: 3 g	Potassium: 993 mg

60. New Orleans Red Beans

Makes 8 servings (Serving size: 1¼ cups)

This vegetarian dish is virtually fat-free and entirely delicious.

1 pound dry red beans
2 quarts water
1½ cups onion, chopped
1 cup celery, chopped
4 bay leaves
1 cup green peppers, chopped
3 tablespoons garlic, chopped
3 tablespoons parsley, chopped
2 teaspoons dried thyme, crushed
1 teaspoon salt
1 teaspoon black pepper

1. Pick through beans to remove bad ones. Rinse beans thoroughly.
2. In large pot, combine beans, water, onion, celery, and bay leaves. Bring to boil. Reduce heat, cover, and cook over low heat for about 1½ hours or until beans are tender. Stir. Mash beans against side of pan.
3. Add green pepper, garlic, parsley, thyme, salt, and black pepper. Cook uncovered over low heat until creamy, about 30 minutes. Remove bay leaves.
4. Serve with hot cooked brown rice, if desired.

EACH SERVING PROVIDES:			
Calories: 171	Cholesterol: 0 mg	Protein: 10 g
Total fat: less than 1 g	Sodium: 285 mg	Carbohydrates: 32 g
Saturated fat: less than 1 g	Total fiber: 7 g	Potassium: 665 mg

61. Zucchini Lasagna

Makes 6 servings (Serving size: 1 piece)

*Say "cheese!" This healthy version of a
favorite comfort food will leave you smiling.*

½ pound lasagna noodles, cooked in
    unsalted water
¾ cup part-skim mozzarella cheese,
    grated
¼ cup Parmesan cheese, grated
1½ cups fat-free cottage cheese
2½ cups no-salt-added tomato sauce
1½ cups raw zucchini, sliced
2 teaspoons basil, dried
2 teaspoons oregano, dried
¼ cup onion, chopped
1 clove garlic
⅛ teaspoon black pepper

1. Preheat oven to 350°F. Spray 9" × 13" baking dish with vegetable oil spray.
2. In small bowl, combine ⅛ cup mozzarella and 1 tablespoon Parmesan cheese. Set aside.
3. In medium bowl, combine remaining mozzarella and Parmesan cheese with all of the cottage cheese.
4. Combine tomato sauce with remaining ingredients. Spread thin layer of tomato sauce in bottom of baking dish. Add a third of noodles in single layer. Spread half of cottage cheese mixture on top. Add layer of zucchini.
5. Repeat layering. Top with noodles, sauce, and reserved cheese mixture. Cover with aluminum foil.
6. Bake for 30 to 40 minutes. Cool for 10 to 15 minutes. Cut into 6 portions.

EACH SERVING PROVIDES:	Calories: 276	Cholesterol: 11 mg	Protein: 19 g
	Total fat: 5 g	Sodium: 380 mg	Carbohydrates: 41 g
	Saturated fat: 2 g	Total fiber: 5 g	Potassium: 561 mg

CHAPTER 13

Bread, Dessert, and Dressing Recipes

Now that you've got some main-dish recipes under your belt, this chapter will help you complete your meals—in a healthy way. Items such as breads, dressings, and desserts are typically considered "extras." They're not a necessary part of your diet, but they do make tasty additions. As long as you keep them light and nutritious, you can still include these items in your meals.

62. Apricot-Orange Bread

Makes 2 loaves (Serving size: one ½-inch slice)

This bread is low in all the right places—saturated fat, cholesterol, and sodium—without losing any taste or texture.

1 package (6 ounces) dried apricots, cut into small pieces

2 cups water

2 tablespoons margarine (trans fat free)

1 cup sugar

1 egg, slightly beaten

1 tablespoon orange peel, freshly grated

3½ cups all-purpose whole-grain flour, sifted

½ cup fat-free dry milk powder

2 teaspoons baking powder

1 teaspoon baking soda

1 teaspoon salt

½ cup orange juice

½ cup pecans, chopped

1. Preheat oven to 350°F. Lightly oil two 9" × 5" loaf pans.
2. Cook apricots in water in covered medium-size saucepan for 10 to 15 minutes or until tender but not mushy. Drain and reserve ¾ cup liquid. Set apricots aside to cool.
3. Cream together margarine and sugar. By hand, beat in egg and orange peel.
4. Sift together flour, dry milk, baking powder, baking soda, and salt. Add to creamed mixture alternately with reserved apricot liquid and orange juice.
5. Stir apricot pieces and pecans into batter.
6. Turn batter into prepared pans.
7. Bake for 40 to 45 minutes.
8. Cool for 5 minutes in pans. Remove from pans and completely cool on wire rack before slicing.

EACH SERVING PROVIDES:	Calories: 97	Cholesterol: 6 mg	Protein: 2 g
	Total fat: 2 g	Sodium: 113 mg	Carbohydrates: 18 g
	Saturated fat: less than 1 g	Total fiber: 1 g	Potassium: 110 mg

63. Apple Coffee Cake

Makes 20 servings (Serving size:
one 3½-inch × 2½-inch piece)

Apples and raisins keep this cake moist—
which means less oil and more health.

5 cups tart apples, cored, peeled,
   chopped
1 cup sugar
1 cup dark raisins
½ cup pecans, chopped
¼ cup vegetable oil
2 teaspoons vanilla
1 egg, beaten
2 cups all-purpose whole-grain flour,
   sifted
1 teaspoon baking soda
2 teaspoons ground cinnamon

1. Preheat oven to 350°F.
2. Lightly oil a 13" × 9" × 2" pan.
3. In large mixing bowl, combine apples
   with sugar, raisins, and pecans. Mix well
   and let stand for 30 minutes.
4. Stir in oil, vanilla, and egg. Sift together
   flour, soda, and cinnamon, and stir into
   apple mixture about a third at a time—
   just enough to moisten dry ingredients.
5. Turn batter into pan. Bake for 35 to 40
   minutes. Cool cake slightly before serving.

EACH SERVING PROVIDES:			
Calories: 196	Cholesterol: 11 mg	Protein: 3 g
Total fat: 8 g	Sodium: 67 mg	Carbohydrates: 31 g
Saturated fat: 1 g	Total fiber: 2 g	Potassium: 136 mg

64. Crunchy Pumpkin Pie

Makes 9 servings (Serving size: 1/9 of 9" pie)

This pie offers a fun, nutritious twist on the classic holiday favorite.

For Crust:
1 cup oats
¼ cup whole-wheat flour
¼ cup ground almonds
2 tablespoons brown sugar
¼ teaspoon salt
3 tablespoons vegetable oil
1 tablespoon water

For Filling:
¼ cup brown sugar, packed
½ teaspoon ground cinnamon
¼ teaspoon ground nutmeg
¼ teaspoon salt
1 egg, beaten
4 teaspoons vanilla
1 cup canned pumpkin
⅔ cup evaporated skim milk

To prepare crust:
1. Preheat oven to 350°F.
2. Mix oats, flour, almonds, brown sugar, and salt in small mixing bowl.
3. Blend oil and water and whisk vigorously.
4. Add oil mixture to dry ingredients and mix.
5. Press into 9" pie pan, and bake for 8 to 10 minutes, or until light brown.

To prepare filling:
6. Mix brown sugar, cinnamon, nutmeg, and salt in bowl.
7. Add egg and vanilla, and mix to blend ingredients. Add pumpkin and milk, and stir to combine.

Putting it together:
8. Pour filling into prepared pie shell.
9. Bake for 45 minutes at 350°F or until done.

EACH SERVING PROVIDES:			
Calories: 169	Cholesterol: 24 mg	Protein: 5 g
Total fat: 7 g	Sodium: 207 mg	Carbohydrates: 22 g
Saturated fat: 1 g	Total fiber: 3 g	Potassium: 223 mg

65. Fresh Salsa

Makes 8 servings (Serving size: ½ cup)

Fresh herbs add plenty of flavor to this salsa—so you use less salt.

6 tomatoes, preferably Roma (or 3
   large tomatoes)
½ medium onion, finely chopped
1 clove garlic, finely minced
2 jalapeño peppers, finely chopped
3 tablespoons cilantro, chopped
Fresh lime juice to taste
⅛ teaspoon oregano, finely crushed
⅛ teaspoon salt
⅛ teaspoon pepper
½ avocado, diced (black skin)

1. Combine all ingredients in glass bowl.
2. Serve immediately or refrigerate and serve within 4 to 5 hours.

EACH SERVING PROVIDES:	Calories: 42	Cholesterol: 0 mg	Protein: 1 g
	Total fat: 2 g	Sodium: 44 mg	Carbohydrates: 7 g
	Saturated fat: less than 1 g	Total fiber: 2 g	Potassium: 337 mg

66. Yogurt Salad Dressing

Makes 8 servings (Serving size: 2 tablespoons)

So easy. So healthy. So good. Try it!

8 ounces fat-free plain yogurt
¼ cup fat-free mayonnaise
2 tablespoons chives, dried
2 tablespoons dill, dried
2 tablespoons lemon juice

Mix all ingredients in bowl and refrigerate.

EACH SERVING PROVIDES:	Calories: 23	Cholesterol: 1 mg	Protein: 2 g
	Total fat: 0 g	Total fiber: 0 g	Carbohydrates: 4 g
	Saturated fat: 0 g	Sodium: 84 mg	Potassium: 104 mg

PART V

WEIGHT MANAGEMENT
AND EXERCISE

CHAPTER 14

Manage Your Weight the Healthy Way

A healthy weight is one that minimizes your risk of illness and disease and falls within the range of weight appropriate for your height. A person may suffer from poor health if overly heavy or overly thin. Each person should find his or her own healthy weight for his or her own body type. It's also important to consult your doctor about your eating habits. Your doctor might even suggest using the services of a registered dietician (RD). For patients with health insurance, many plans cover consultations with RDs if requested by a physician. For those without insurance, many hospitals offer classes in "healthful cooking and eating" and lowering cholesterol at very low cost. This is great!

67. Understand Your Body Composition

Your body is composed of fat mass and lean body mass. Together, this is referred to as your body composition. Ideally, you want to keep the percentage of fat quite a bit lower than the percentage of nonfat mass. (Your nonfat mass includes your bones, organs, and muscle.) And, if you decide to lose weight, you want to lose fat, not valuable muscle tissue that gives you strength and support.

Researchers have found that the amount of body fat is not the only factor that is important. What is equally, if not more, significant is where the fat is deposited on your body. Studies show that people whose bodies store fat around the abdominal area, also referred to as an "apple shaped" body, are at higher risk of heart disease, stroke, high blood pressure, and Type 2 diabetes than those people who are more "pear shaped" and carry their excess fat around their hips and thighs.

To determine whether or not you have abdominal obesity, you need to measure your waist circumference. For purposes of this measurement, your waist is considered to be halfway between the lowest rib and the top of your hipbone, measured when you are upright and your trunk is perpendicular to the floor. A waist circumference of greater than forty inches for men, or greater than thirty-five inches for women, may indicate a higher risk of heart disease.

68. Calculate Your Body Mass Index (BMI)

Another method to assess whether your weight may put you at risk is to calculate your body mass index (BMI). The BMI expresses weight relative to height. It provides a general guideline to check whether you are in a healthy weight range. A high BMI score may indicate increased risks for heart disease, high blood pressure, diabetes, and high cholesterol. BMI guidelines are not accurate for estimating risks for people who are healthy at higher weight levels, such as muscular competitive athletes or pregnant women. These guidelines also do not apply to growing children or frail and sedentary older adults.

There are many websites through which you can determine your BMI, including the Centers for Disease Control and Prevention at *www.cdc.gov*. If your BMI is greater than 25, you fall into the category of overweight. A BMI between 18.5 and 24.9 is considered a healthy weight. If your BMI score is less than 18.5, you are considered to be underweight.

69. Recognize the Causes of Weight Gain

In simplistic terms, one can say that the cause of weight gain is taking in excess calories. But this does not take into full consideration the complex social factors that make it difficult to live an active lifestyle, to enjoy wholesome fresh foods, and to separate emotional factors from the need to eat. Furthermore, as researchers learn more and more about the differences among people's metabolic profiles, it seems that depending on the types of foods that are consumed, some people are more prone to gain weight easily and to have a more difficult time of losing it. The overall picture is complex, but a few simple factors play key roles.

Emotional Overeating

Many people overeat in response to cues that are completely unrelated to hunger. Stress can play a role, as can environmental factors in the home. For example, if your parents rewarded you with a food treat when you accomplished tasks, you may continue to give yourself this type of treat when you finish something as an adult. Similarly, if food was used to cope with emotions rather than discussing, facing, or experiencing emotions, it can continue to play that role in adult life.

Keeping a journal can be helpful for people who find that they eat in response to these types of emotional cues, rather than to true feelings of hunger. In the journal, you can record what triggered an eating episode, what you were thinking and feeling at the time, and what feelings you were avoiding by eating. This process may be very revealing as you start to unravel some of your more unconscious eating behaviors that lead to overconsumption of food.

Eating Highly Refined, Processed Foods

Another factor that can contribute to overeating is choosing foods that are highly refined and processed. In this case, the overeating often occurs in response to genuine hunger cues. For example, breads and pastas that are made with enriched flour rather than with whole grains lack fiber that provides important feelings of fullness and satiety. Drinking juices instead of eating fruits is also another missed opportunity to eat fiber-rich foods.

Fiber, both soluble and insoluble, is critically important to health. Not only does it provide roughage that is good for digestion, but it also lowers cholesterol levels and makes you feel full. It truly is hard to overeat when your meals are filled with wholesome fresh fruits, vegetables, and whole grains.

Lack of Physical Activity

Living an active lifestyle in today's technology-driven world is a challenge. It is actually much easier to live a sedentary life today than it is to live an active life. Many of us start our day by traveling to work or to school via cars or buses. We spend much of our day seated in chairs with few breaks from our sitting lifestyle. When we return home at the end of the day, we are tired and hungry and the last thing we feel like doing is "exercising."

Without a conscious effort to move, it's actually quite easy to be completely inactive all day long. When this lack of movement is combined with overconsumption of foods, it's easy to see how the combination can quickly add to increased weight gain.

Loss of Lean Body Mass

An aspect of the picture that affects metabolism and activity levels is the natural decline in lean body mass that occurs with aging. After the age of thirty-five, both men and women lose approximately one-third to one-half pound of muscle each year. If your total weight is not changing, this means that this loss of lean body mass has been replaced by an equivalent gain of fat mass. Although your weight may not have changed, the difference between these two types of tissues is extremely significant from the point of view of weight management.

The loss of lean body mass means your body is composed of less of the metabolically more active tissue as well as a decrease in the muscle that provides strength to move and accomplish physical tasks. So not only is the body burning fewer calories even at rest, but it also becomes more tired and less capable of doing things such as walking up the stairs, running after children, and lifting and carrying grocery bags.

This is the beginning of a cycle of reduced daily physical activity that leads to even more fat gain. Over time, the ratio of fat becomes high and the amount of lean is low. The older adult may no longer have the strength to even climb a flight of stairs or get up and move around at all, and the pounds can easily add up.

70. Follow Strategies for Successful Weight Management

Managing your weight is part of a healthy lifestyle. To achieve success, it's best to make changes gradually and to have realistic expectations. The following tips can help you get started:

- Examine your eating habits. Are you meeting the necessary requirements?
- Portion size matters. Learn what healthy single servings of food should be, and adjust your portion sizes.
- Get active each and every day. Every movement counts.
- Incorporate strength or weight training to increase your lean body mass.

As you improve your daily habits, instead of focusing on changes in your scale weight, notice changes in how you feel. Do you have more energy? Are you feeling stronger? Are you sleeping better at night?

If you're the type who needs a goal in the form of a number, such as weight, to keep you motivated, think about measuring your progress in other ways. Get your cholesterol and blood sugar levels tested. Check whether your resting heart rate and blood pressure levels are going down. Most importantly, know you're doing the best that you can for your long-term well-being.

CHAPTER 15

Get Active

Along with eating a balanced diet of minimally processed whole foods, being active on most days of the week is critical to creating healthy cholesterol levels. Getting active for health does not mean spending hours at the gym. In fact, you never even have to go to the gym to get the amount of exercise that is proven to improve your health. This chapter will give you the knowledge of why physical activity is beneficial and how you can get moving to enjoy those results.

71. Learn the Benefits of Movement

Physical inactivity is a major risk factor for heart disease. The heart is a muscle that benefits from regular use to keep it and the circulatory system healthy. When a person is inactive, the heart muscle is weaker. With each beat, an unfit heart muscle pumps a lower volume of blood than a stronger, more fit heart.

Because less blood is pumped, the heart has to beat more frequently in order to ensure adequate circulation of blood around the body. This more rapid heart rate can also result in an increase in blood pressure over time, causing stiffness and hardening of the arteries and impacting the health of the circulatory system. In contrast, when the heart is strong and healthy, stroke volume is strong. The heart rate is slower, and a more healthy tone is maintained in the arterial walls.

Increasing physical activity leads to an increase in the levels of HDL, or good cholesterol. This change is independent of any weight loss that may also occur as increased activity burns up more calories. Physical activity also lowers LDL and triglyceride levels.

Studies show that regular physical activity not only lowers bad cholesterol and triglycerides and increases good cholesterol, but that it also reduces risk of death from all causes, reduces feelings of depression and anxiety, and helps build and maintain healthy bones, muscles, and joints.

72. Discover How Much Activity Is Enough

According to guidelines issued by the U.S. Surgeon General, the U.S. Department of Health and Human Services, and the National Heart, Lung, and Blood

Institute, the minimum amount of activity for health includes the following factors:

- Should continue for at least 30 minutes total
- Can be accumulated in bouts as short as 8 to 10 minutes
- Should be of moderate intensity, such as brisk walking
- Should occur on most, preferably all, days of the week
- Should include some resistance exercise and stretching during the week

The guidelines also note that more activity and a higher intensity will provide greater health and fitness benefits. The general guidelines listed above set forth minimum amounts of activity necessary to enjoy health benefits. Clearly, this level of exercise will not prepare you to run a marathon or to climb Mount Everest, but such events may not be among your immediate goals. You may simply want to feel better and know you are doing something good for your health. The message for you is loud and clear—with moderate amounts of physical activity on a regular basis, you can achieve this goal.

73. Work Activity into Your Lifestyle

Many of us are so conditioned into thinking that exercise means going to the gym that we forget that everyday life presents us with numerous opportunities to get active during the day. If you have time to go to the gym, that's fantastic. But if you don't, do not despair. You can create more movement opportunities during your day that make a difference. Look for every opportunity to be active.

Here are some examples of lifestyle activity:

- Walk to run an errand in the neighborhood, rather than taking a car.
- Play outdoor games with children instead of watching television together.
- Park farther away from the shop.
- Get off the train or bus one stop early and walk the rest of the way.
- Carry your groceries to your car or load them into your car yourself.
- Wash your car instead of taking it to the car wash.
- Rake leaves instead of using a leaf blower.
- Get up to switch appliances on or off instead of always using a remote control.
- Ride a bicycle for transportation instead of driving a car.
- Do some vigorous house cleaning, such as vacuuming, sweeping, or mopping.
- If you live or work in an office building, take the stairs (up!), adding one floor each week.
- Take an active vacation that involves hiking, camping, biking, or horseback riding instead of lolling on a cruise boat or at a beach and eating.
- If you have a yard, gardening is an excellent form of exercise.

Be creative. Find more and more ways that you can move during your day. These activities all add up and make a difference. For example, according to estimates for a 150-pound person, standing up for three ten-minute phone calls will burn twenty calories. In contrast, sitting for thirty minutes during those three phone calls burns only four calories. Simply by standing for those brief intervals, you have created a sixteen-calorie deficit. While sixteen calories may not seem like much, when it is repeated hour after hour, day after day, it and other small actions start to mean the difference between unwanted pounds and maintaining your ideal weight. If you added walking or pacing to your phone calls, it would even provide greater benefits.

74. Walk Your Way to a Healthy Heart

One of the best forms of exercise that provides a healthful challenge for the human body is walking. It is economical, easy to fit into your day, bears a low risk of injury, and is effective in improving health. Numerous studies show that people who walk regularly have less risk of death or disability from disease. Studies have also shown that people who participate in regular walking programs have higher levels of HDL cholesterol, lower levels of total and LDL cholesterol, and lower levels of triglycerides or blood fats.

Try a Walking Program

Before you get started with any exercise program, it is a good idea to check with your health care provider. If you are apparently healthy and under the age of sixty-five, then you are likely to be fine with a moderate exercise program. If, however, you are older or have any known chronic conditions such as arthritis, diabetes, or heart disease, work out an appropriate program with your health care provider.

Get the Right Footwear

Take the time to find a comfortable, sturdy shoe that fits the needs of your foot and provides good arch support. Shoe technology these days is quite sophisticated. Go to a reputable athletic footwear store that allows returns if the shoe is not a good fit for you.

Buy shoe inserts. Today's shoes do not come with insoles that last as long as the outer part of the shoe. Yet the cushioning that provides you with support is essential to keep you comfortable and to prevent injury. When you purchase your shoes, ask the salesperson to also help you to find an appropriate insole. This will make a tremendous difference in your long-term comfort.

Dress the Part

As far as sportswear for walking, you want to wear fabrics that breathe, such as cotton or polyester blends. Many modern fabrics also feature wicking qualities that actually draw your perspiration away from your skin. This can definitely enhance your walking comfort. Women who need the extra support should wear an athletic sports bra. Comfort is your primary objective.

Sun protection is also important. Be sure to wear sunscreen. A hat is also a good idea to protect your face. Depending on how sensitive you are to sun exposure, you may want to purchase a hat that also shields the back of your neck. Sunglasses provide coverage for your eyes.

Consider a Pedometer

A pedometer is a great tool to measure your progress and keep you motivated. Studies show that if you take 10,000 steps on most days of the week, you will realize many health benefits. (This equates to about five miles a day.)

Furthermore, if you take 12,000 to 15,000 steps per day, it can help you accomplish your weight loss goals.

The steps the pedometer measures do not have to be performed at a particular intensity level or for a specific duration. What they represent is that you have maintained a level of daily activity that contributes to your health.

75. Get Started on a Walking Program

When you begin, start out at a comfortable pace. Let your arms hang naturally at your sides so they swing rhythmically with each step. Be sure to stand tall and maintain good posture. After about five minutes of walking, if you enjoy performing some stretches to make your walk more comfortable, you can.

Walking Technique

Posture is the most important aspect of walking technique. Stand tall with your ears aligned with your shoulders, arms at your sides, shoulders aligned with hips, and abdominal muscles slightly pulled in to actively support your lower back. If you want to increase the intensity of your walk, bend your elbows and swing your arms more vigorously. Take more steps, rather than longer strides. Keep your focus ahead to maintain good posture. Let your heel strike first and push forward through the ball of your foot. Keep your elbows in and avoid swinging your arms across your body.

Walking Cooldown

After you finish the brisker portion of your walk, take time to slowly bring your body back to the way it felt when you began. Gradually slow back down to the comfortable pace you started out with. By the time you stop walking, your breathing should be relaxed and your heart rate should be calm. You only need to spend a few minutes on your walking cooldown, but be sure to take this time.

After your walk is a great time to include some final stretches. Unlike the beginning of your walk, your muscles are warm and ready to enjoy a long stretch. Good stretches to perform include shoulder rolls for the neck and shoulders, a standing calf stretch for the back of the lower leg, hamstring stretch for the back of the upper leg, standing side stretch for the side of the torso, and standing cat stretch to release the lower back. Breathe deeply, and hold each stretch anywhere from twenty to thirty seconds.

PART VI

OTHER WAYS TO MANAGE CHOLESTEROL

CHAPTER 16

Stress Management

Stress is a daily aspect of modern living. It can keep you motivated and even save your life. If unmanaged, however, stress can kill you. Excess stress weakens the immune system. Furthermore, stress can make any disease condition worse. In this chapter, we will discover what stress is, how stress contributes to heart disease, how you can identify stress, and what steps you can take to reduce stress and restore balance to your life.

76. Know What Stress Is

Stress is a natural physiological response to something that triggers a feeling of fear or threat. This response, called "fight or flight," is designed to help us survive life-threatening situations. The natural chemical response that affects your mind and body is like a miracle drug that can help save your life in the face of a dangerous emergency.

The Stress Response

The body's response to stress is stimulated by stress hormones, like adrenaline and cortisol, released by your body to prepare you for action. Among other things, these stress hormones do the following:

- Increase your heart rate and blood pressure to pump an extra burst of oxygen-rich blood around your body so you can get moving.
- Stop the flow of blood to your digestive system and skin by constricting arteries.
- Increase blood flow to the brain and muscles by relaxing arteries.
- Increase perspiration to cool the body.
- Speed up breathing rate and open bronchial tubes to draw more oxygen-rich air into the lungs.

When you look at all of these changes, it's easy to see how this chemically induced state of emergency preparedness is extremely useful in life-threatening situations.

How Stress Causes Harm

Stress can be harmful to health if it mounts to levels at which you feel that you can no longer cope. This usually occurs after stress levels have remained high over a prolonged period of time.

Physical and mental symptoms of excessive stress include high blood pressure, rapid pulse, chronic muscle tension, headaches, digestive problems, irritability, depression, anxiety, loss of ability to concentrate, altered sleeping or eating habits, and increased use of drugs or alcohol. High stress can even increase the risk of a heart attack. Understanding stress and having skills to manage stress effectively, therefore, is important to your overall health and wellness.

77. Learn about Stress and Heart Disease

The American Heart Association does not include stress as one of the leading risk factors for heart disease. However, this may have more to do with the difficulty of teasing out stress from other risk factors than with the fact that stress does not contribute to risk of heart disease. In other words, it is difficult to prove that stress is an independent risk factor given that it also contributes to other behaviors, such as smoking, physical inactivity, and overeating, that all undermine health. The American Heart Association, however, does note that individual responses to stress may be a contributing factor to heart disease risk.

Stress and Heart Function

After studying the long-term effects of stress, some researchers believe that prolonged stress can cause damage to blood vessels. A 2002 study reported that mental stress causes the inner lining of the blood vessels (the endothelial lining) to constrict, which can increase the risk of sudden cardiac death. This constriction leads to endothelial dysfunction, a precursor to the development of atherosclerosis.

did you know . . . ?

For people with diabetes, stress can have a detrimental effect on management of blood glucose levels. While individual responses vary, people with Type 2 diabetes find that stress often increases blood glucose levels. Since high levels of blood glucose can also damage the health of blood vessels, it is particularly important for people with diabetes to effectively manage stress.

Over time, the blood vessels lose their ability to dilate effectively until the blood vessels cannot respond appropriately to changes in blood demands. For example, constricted arteries would be unable to provide an increased blood flow to meet the needs of working muscles in the legs or to meet the increased demands of blood flow to a heart that is pumping more vigorously to support physical activity.

Stress and Blood Cholesterol Levels

Studies show that long-term stress is associated with elevated blood cholesterol levels. In these studies, however, it is difficult to isolate the exact cause. Some scientists theorize that stress indirectly causes high cholesterol by providing a fertile ground for bad health habits. For example, people who feel highly stressed are likely to overeat high-fat foods, smoke, and drink excess amounts of alcohol. Other researchers believe that the chemical changes that are part of the stress response may play a role in affecting blood fats and blood sugars, vessel health, and heart function.

78. Identify Stress in Your Life

Some people thrive in situations that make others miserably tense and anxious. For example, you may hate meeting deadlines, while a friend works productively under that type of pressure. If you are frequently rushed or competitive and feel overwhelmed by this, or you let small frustrations get to you, or you find it hard to forget your worries and relax, reducing these stressors will most likely improve your health. At the same time, you can certainly make your life more enjoyable.

Other types of stress are not caused by your attitude, but are rather the product of a busy life. For example, if you are driving in heavy traffic and someone quickly cuts in front of you, that is a stressful situation. You have a legitimate fear for your safety as a car accident could result. Your reaction, however, does not require you to burn off any physical energy. Rather, you remain seated in your car. You are likely to tighten your muscles and experience feelings of tension and anxiety as your body undergoes the physiological and biochemical changes associated with the "fight or flight" response.

Often, when you feel "stressed out," it is a generalized feeling of stress. If you take a moment to examine your situation, however, you will find that your feelings are actually the cumulative result of numerous individual pressures that have finally reached the boiling point. One of the first steps to learn how to manage stress effectively is to identify these individual pressures—the types of things in your life that cause you stress. Your awareness is the first step.

The next time you start to feel overwhelmed and stressed out, explore these feelings in greater depth. Ask yourself the following questions to determine what is causing these emotions:

- Am I overcommitted?
- Am I taking care of others and neglecting my own self-care?
- Am I trying to accomplish everything on my own without asking for any support from anyone else?
- Are my expectations unrealistic?
- What is going on in my life right now that gives me a sense of struggle?

If you are the type of person who finds it helpful to keep a journal, try to record things that trigger your stress. Write down what happened, what you were thinking or feeling, and how you reacted physically. This can give you valuable insight into the cumulative triggers you face throughout the day.

79. Use Strategies to Deal with Stress

It's important to make time to learn stress management skills and relaxation techniques. Learning how to manage stress or how to eliminate some of the stressors in your life is important when it comes to keeping your immune system strong, reducing your risk of illness, and improving your feelings of well-being.

Identify Priorities and Manage Time Effectively

Time management is a critical skill to develop in order to successfully manage stress. Everyone has the same number of hours in the day. Some people, however, are more effective managers of their time and priorities. To get organized, first identify your priorities. Next, make a realistic plan for how long it will take to get things done. Do the best that you can, and remember to also leave time for yourself.

Rely on Social Support

Social support is a very important factor in effective stress management. Friends and family can help you to talk over troublesome topics and help you keep your perspective. Take time to make friends and to maintain relationships. Even a cherished pet can provide you with companionship and dispel feelings of loneliness and isolation.

If you feel that you need more support, go ahead and ask for help from others in your home, workplace, or community. Your employer may have an employee assistance program that can provide you with confidential counseling. Your church or community center may also have helpful resources.

Express Yourself Without Anger

Remember that people who get angry easily are much more likely to die from a heart attack. If you find that you are often irritated or annoyed, learn constructive methods to deal with disagreeable situations. Learn more effective communication skills to defuse conflicts. Make sure that you are not allowing resentment to build up inside you. Over time, denial of anger can lead to unhealthy blowups or chronic negative feelings. The healthiest approach is to learn how to effectively express your feelings in positive and constructive ways.

It may help to remember some simple alternatives to becoming angry or frustrated in stressful situations. If possible, leave the scene of a stressful situation before it gets to you. Talk to someone you trust about how you feel, or take some time on your own to brainstorm nonstressful ways to respond to a stressful issue. Most importantly, remember to breathe deeply, and ask yourself, "In the scheme of things, does this really matter?"

Make Time for Self-Care

One of the biggest contributors to feelings of stress is the sense that life is out of control. To avoid this, make time for yourself. You deserve time for your own self-care. For one thing, it supports your health, which in turn helps you to better support all the people around you that you care about. Take a moment to identify things that you enjoy, that bring you pleasure, and that are fun and restorative. Make it a point to incorporate these activities into your schedule.

80. Restore Your Health Through Relaxation

One of the easiest ways to achieve relaxation is to engage in deep, mindful breathing exercises. This can help to trigger the relaxation response. This type of exercise is easy to learn, quick to perform, and requires no equipment. As you continue to explore other methods of relaxation, use the following breathing exercise to help you ease tensions and restore your sense of balance and calm. It will do the health of your body, mind, and spirit a world of good.

Try a simple breathing exercise. The following is an excellent introduction to relaxation and to meditation techniques. It increases self and body awareness. A two- to three-minute "breathing break" during the day is very restorative. To perform this simple exercise, sit or lie comfortably with your hands resting in your lap. Relax your muscles and close your eyes.

Make no effort to control your breath—simply breathe naturally. As you breathe in and out, focus your attention on the breath and how the body moves with each inhalation and exhalation.

Take a few moments to focus inward. Notice the movement of your body as you breathe. Observe your inhalation and exhalation. Pay particular attention to how the breath moves your body. Observe your chest, shoulders, rib cage, and belly. Notice subtleties such as whether the chest or belly rises with inhalation and how your body responds to exhalation. Don't try to control your breath, simply focus your attention on it. This singular focus brings you into the present moment and into the immediate experience of your body. It often results in slower, deeper breaths that further relax your body. Continue for two to three minutes and then gently open your eyes. Over time, you can lengthen the period of relaxation, if you prefer.

CHAPTER 17

Live Smoke-Free

Smoking cigarettes greatly increases your risk of having a heart attack or stroke. Chemicals such as nicotine in cigarettes damage the lining of blood vessels and reduce HDL, or good cholesterol. In spite of the fact that nicotine is highly addictive, you can apply any of several strategies to successfully kick your smoking habit. The good news is that within minutes of your last cigarette, your body starts to change for the better.

81. Face the Harmful Effects of Smoking

When compared to nonsmokers, smokers have twice the risk of having a heart attack or stroke. Furthermore, smokers who have a heart attack are much more likely to die. Smoking increases the risk of sudden cardiac death.

Cigarette smoking specifically harms the heart and circulatory system in a number of ways, including the following:

- Damaging the lining of the arteries
- Decreasing HDL cholesterol
- Accelerating plaque formation by increasing oxidation of LDL cholesterol
- Escalating heart rate and blood pressure by narrowing the arteries
- Reducing the amount of available oxygen in the bloodstream by increasing levels of carbon monoxide
- Raising the likelihood of blood clot formation

For the nonsmoker, secondhand smoke poses the same risks as inhaled smoke pose to the smoker because the lethal chemicals are in the smoke itself. Therefore, passive smoking or simply breathing smoke-filled air draws those same chemicals into the lungs and bloodstream.

According to research studies, nonsmokers exposed to environmental tobacco smoke were at a 25 percent higher relative risk of developing heart disease than nonsmokers not exposed to environmental tobacco smoke. According to the American Heart Association, approximately 37,000 to 40,000 nonsmokers die each year from cardiovascular disease (CVD) resulting from exposure to passive tobacco smoke. Accordingly, the 2002 American Heart Association Guidelines for Primary Prevention of Cardiovascular Disease and Stroke recommend no exposure to tobacco smoke to prevent heart attack and stroke. While it may be impossible to completely prevent exposure to second-hand smoke, you will benefit from avoiding it as much as you can.

82. Look at the Benefits of Quitting

The health benefits of kicking the smoking habit truly start right away. Within twenty minutes of your last cigarette, nicotine is no longer causing constriction of blood vessels. As a result, your blood pressure decreases, your heart rate slows, and the temperature of your hands and feet rises as circulation improves. Within eight hours of your last cigarette, carbon monoxide levels drop in the bloodstream, and oxygen levels increase. Within twenty-four hours, the chances of having a heart attack are reduced. Within forty-eight hours, nerve endings begin to regenerate, and your sense of smell and taste start to return.

During the first year of not smoking, your body continues to heal itself from the stress of absorbing all the cigarette toxins. Coughing, sinus congestion, fatigue, and shortness of breath start to fade as the strength of the lungs is restored. After a smoke-free year, the increased risk from smoking is cut in half. With each passing year, the risk continues to diminish.

Another great benefit of quitting is that you will save quite a bit of money by giving up the cigarette habit. Your savings come mostly from the fact that you no longer need to buy cigarettes. Since smoking increases your risk for so many diseases, you also save money by staying healthy and not creating huge medical bills.

83. Make a Plan to Quit Smoking

Many smokers try to quit multiple times before they eventually succeed, but thorough preparation can increase your odds of achieving a smoke-free future. The federal government provides resources to assist people. In a program set forth on the website www.smokefree.gov, the preparatory phase consists of five steps that can be remembered by the acronym "**START**." The five steps include the following:

S = Set a quit date.
T = Tell family, friends, and coworkers that you plan to quit.
A = Anticipate and plan for the challenges that you will face.
R = Remove tobacco products from your home, car, and work.
T = Talk to your health care provider.

Set a Quit Date

Once you have your mind made up that the benefits of not smoking far outweigh the risks of smoking, then you are ready to set a quit date. Be sure that you are genuinely ready to make this commitment before you decide upon your quit date. Choose a specific day at least two weeks in advance. This gives you plenty of time to prepare, without losing your motivation to quit.

Tell Others Your Plan

Social support is the single most important factor in determining whether you are successful in changing poor habits into good ones. The help of your family and friends makes changing any behavioral pattern much easier.

Share your quitting plans with those who are close to you to solicit their support.

The National Cancer Institute offers a smoking cessation guide with several helpful tips for developing your support system. First of all, the institute advises you to be sure to remind friends that your moods may change. Let them know that the longer you go without cigarettes, the sooner you will return to your old self. Also, if you have a friend or family member close to you who also smokes, see if he or she is interested in quitting with you. If not, ask him or her not to smoke around you. Seek out an ex-smoker to give you encouragement and advice during your tough moments.

Anticipate Challenges and Plan Ahead

Most people tend to form habitual patterns of smoking, such as immediately after a meal or when enjoying an alcoholic drink. These are the times that will present you with the strongest cravings. In addition to emotional cravings, most smokers also experience withdrawal symptoms including mood swings, feelings of irritability and depression, anxiety or restlessness, insomnia, headaches, difficulty concentrating, and increased hunger.

These symptoms are worst the first few weeks, and they are extremely powerful during the first week of quitting. To help manage the cravings, use the time before you quit to concentrate on the moments you observe that you want a cigarette most. Note when you have a cigarette and how you are feeling at the time. Then consider alternative ways to cope with those feelings and alternative activities during those times. For example, instead of having a cigarette after a meal, chew gum, drink water, squirt your mouth with breath spray, or brush your teeth. Be proactive in planning these alternatives, and buy the gum, breath spray, or whatever else you will need before you get to your scheduled quitting day.

Remove Cigarettes and Other Tobacco Products

Take a look around you. Take note of all the visual cues that support your smoking so you can start eliminating them from your environment. For example, throw out ashtrays, lighters, and matches. Remove the lighter in your car. Clean your home, office, and car by using air freshener and ridding all remnants of cigarette smoke. Make an appointment with your dentist to have your teeth cleaned and polished.

just the facts

Be especially careful to not smoke when you are using one of the nicotine replacement therapies. Keep in mind that these products are providing nicotine to your body and that it is possible to overdose. Be aware of the signs of nicotine poisoning, which can include severe headaches, weakness, dizziness, nausea, vomiting, diarrhea, cold sweats, blurred vision, hearing difficulties, or mental confusion.

Talk to Your Health Care Provider

Be sure to discuss your quitting plan with your health care provider. If you are taking any prescription medications, find out how your drug therapy may be affected by changing your smoking habits.

Nicotine is powerfully addictive. There are medications that can help you avoid withdrawal symptoms. Enlist the support of your health care provider, and discuss your options together.

84. Get Help with Quitting Smoking

Many products exist today to aid the transition to a smoke-free life. Studies show that people who use nicotine replacement therapy are almost twice as successful as those who do not. Some smoking cessation aids are available over the counter; others require a prescription.

Nicotine Gum, Lozenges, and Patches

Nicotine gum, lozenges, and patches are available over the counter at your local pharmacy or grocery store. These products provide a low level of nicotine, without the accompanying toxins that come from smoking, to help you overcome the withdrawal symptoms.

The most common mistake people make with these products is not using enough. Do not skimp or underestimate the amount that you think you will need. Follow the directions on the package, and do not forget to continue to use your product. Over time, you can reduce the amount that you use. Always keep some of the medication around to help you avoid cravings.

Nicotine Inhalers and Nasal Sprays

Nicotine inhalers and nasal sprays both require a prescription from your doctor. Nasal sprays can provide immediate relief. Furthermore, sprays come in different concentrations so that you can reduce the amount of nicotine you put into your system over time.

Nicotine inhalers deliver nicotine into your system in much the same manner as cigarettes. For example, when you use a nicotine inhaler, you breathe the medication in through a mouthpiece. The nicotine is absorbed through the mouth's lining.

Bupropion Pills

In contrast to the nicotine replacement therapies, bupropion pills do not contain nicotine. Bupropion pills are an antidepressant that help to reduce withdrawal symptoms and cigarette cravings. If you and your physician think this would be a good approach for you, you can even start taking the pill before your quit date.

This medication does require a prescription, however, and as it does have side effects, it is not appropriate for everyone. Medical experts recommend that pregnant women, people with eating disorders or who experience seizures, and people who drink heavily not use this medication.

Chantix is now the preferred prescription drug for smoking cessation. It is more effective than bupropion with fewer side effects.

85. Avoid Relapsing into Smoking

Quitting the cigarette habit is among the most challenging tasks that you will face. Be prepared, particularly in the first few days and weeks, to have alternate plans to keep you busy and to help you avoid dwelling on your urges to have a cigarette. Be especially prepared for those times of day when you are accustomed to sitting back and lighting up. Here are some suggestions for other ways to use this time:

- Take a walk.
- Have some healthy snacks around to chew on.
- Drink lots of water.
- Chew gum or suck on candy.
- Perform breathing exercises.
- Pick up a craft such as knitting or crocheting to keep your hands busy.
- Enjoy a hot bath and listen to music.
- Spend time with or call supportive friends.
- Take time out to enjoy a good book.

Certain pastimes should also be avoided in these first few critical weeks. To help you stay away from these triggers:

- Limit intake of caffeinated and alcoholic beverages.
- Pass up invitations to spend time with people who smoke.
- If you must spend time with smokers, immediately inform them that you have quit.
- Practice refusing the offer of a cigarette so you will be prepared with your reply.
- Steer clear of places where other people are smoking.
- Eat regularly, and include snacks to avoid extreme feelings of hunger.
- Try not to push yourself into feeling overly tired.
- Pamper and spoil yourself, and indulge in other pleasures.

- Surround yourself with supportive friends and family, and stay away from circumstances that inflame strong emotions such as anger, resentment, or loneliness.

When a strong smoking urge strikes, immediately engage in one of your alternate activities. Continue to remind yourself of all the great benefits that you will experience once you have quit your habit.

CHAPTER 18

Drug Therapy

Reducing your risk of CVD, disability, and death requires that you make a commitment to support and enhance healthful living. Medications support this process. Drugs can be valuable tools to help you achieve optimal health. For some people, drug therapy to manage lipid levels is the best short-term action, until lifestyle changes have time to improve cardiovascular health. For others, drug therapy is the only way to address genetic tendencies toward unhealthy lipid levels.

86. Consider Using Drugs to Treat High Cholesterol

This chapter provides an overview of the various drugs frequently prescribed to manage lipids, such as statins, bile acid sequestrants, nicotinic acid, and fibrates, separately or in combination. As you read about side effects, keep in mind that pharmaceuticals can be very beneficial. Do not become alarmed by precautions and necessary safeguards; it's important to be informed to make intelligent choices.

According to federal government guidelines and American Heart Association recommendations, drug therapy should always be accompanied by health-enhancing lifestyle changes. In fact, studies show that drug therapy is more effective when used together with lifestyle changes to achieve healthy cholesterol levels and reduce the risk of heart attack and stroke. All therapies, therefore, need to be considered in the context of your lifestyle.

When you incorporate a multipronged approach, you get results more quickly, you are able to reduce your medication levels sooner, and you will feel the improvements in your health more rapidly.

87. Do Your Research on Statins

For physicians, statins (known formally as HMG-CoA reductase inhibitors) are usually the drugs of choice for improving cholesterol levels. The primary goal of all lipid therapy is reduction of LDL cholesterol. Since statins lower LDL cholesterol more than any other type of drug, physicians typically consider statins first.

Statins accomplish this reduction of blood LDL by two different processes. First, they inhibit a liver enzyme, HMG-CoA reductase, needed to manufacture cholesterol, thereby decreasing the amount of cholesterol manufactured by the liver and the amount of LDL the liver can produce. Since the liver needs cholesterol, the liver removes more cholesterol from the bloodstream in the form of LDL to replace what it has been inhibited from manufacturing.

Types and Usage

Types of statins include lovastatin, simvastatin, pravastatin, fluvastatin, atorvastatin, and rosuvastatin. These are marketed under the brand names Mevacor, Zocor, Pravachol, Lescol, Lipitor, and Crestor, respectively. Since the body makes more cholesterol at night than during the day, patients are usually directed to take statins in a single dose at the evening meal or at bedtime.

Typically, statins impact cholesterol levels within four to six weeks. After about six to eight weeks, your health care provider will retest your cholesterol levels to determine the effectiveness of the statin therapy and whether the dose requires adjustment.

Side Effects

Most people do not have serious side effects when taking statins. Some people may experience constipation, stomach pain, cramps, or gas. These symptoms are usually mild to moderate, however, and they go away over time. More serious side effects can result from an increase in liver enzymes that can lead to liver toxicity. Because of this risk, it's important to have your liver function tested periodically while you are on statin therapy. People with active chronic liver disease should not take statins.

Another serious side effect comes from statin myopathy. Muscle soreness, pain, and weakness may occur. In extreme cases, muscle cells can break down and release the protein myoglobin into the blood. Myoglobin in the urine can contribute to impaired kidney function, eventually leading to kidney failure. The risk of this occurring is increased when statins are taken in combination with any of the following drugs: the cholesterol-lowering gemfibrozil (brand name Lopid); the antibiotics erythromycin (Erythrocin) and clarithromycin (Biaxin); the antifungals ketoconazole (Nizoral) and itraconazole (Sporanox); the antidepressant nefazodone (Serzone); the immunosuppressive cyclosporine (Sandimmune or Neoral); and niacin.

Contact your health care provider immediately if you experience any adverse side effects. Avoid consuming grapefruit juice, grapefruits, or tangelos (a hybrid grapefruit) when you are taking statins, as these fruits can impact how the drug is metabolized. Grapefruits contain a chemical that affects certain digestive enzymes as drugs are broken down in the intestinal tract and liver.

88. Learn about Bile Acid Sequestrants or Resins

Bile acid sequestrants, also referred to as bile acid resins, reduce LDL cholesterol by binding with cholesterol-rich bile acids in the intestines to facilitate their elimination from the body through the stool. Think back to the overview in Chapter 1 of the liver's role in the cholesterol-manufacturing process. The liver uses cholesterol to manufacture bile acids, a digestive enzyme that breaks down fats. Bile acid sequestrants cause the body to eliminate bile acids in the intestines. Since the body needs bile acids to digest fats, the liver must manufacture more bile acids to replace those eliminated by the drug. The liver uses up its available cholesterol to make more acids, thus making less cholesterol available for release into the bloodstream. Bile acid sequestrants can reduce LDL cholesterol levels from 10 to 20 percent.

Types and Usage

Types of bile acid resins include cholestyramine (brand name Prevalite or Questran), and colestipol (Colestid). Cholestyramine and colestipol are often taken as powders that must be mixed with water or fruit juice and taken either once or twice a day with meals. Both drugs are also available as tablets. There is also a newer bile acid sequestrant, called colesevelam. Use of colesevelam has reduced LDL cholesterol by as much as 12 to 18 percent and is also easier to administer and better tolerated than some of the other products.

Side Effects

The principle side effects with the use of bile acid resins have to do with digestion. This type of drug can cause a variety of gastrointestinal problems, such as constipation, bloating, fullness, nausea, abdominal pain, and gas. Drinking lots of water and eating high-fiber foods can help with these side effects. Physicians generally do not prescribe bile acid resins to people with a history of constipation problems.

Taking bile acids can also inhibit the absorption of certain nutrients from foods and of other medications. Physicians recommend that you take other prescription medications at least one hour before or at least four to six hours after the bile acid sequestrant.

89. Get Educated about Nicotinic Acid

Nicotinic acid, known as niacin or vitamin B_3, is being recommended more often as a way to reduce total blood cholesterol, LDL cholesterol, and triglyceride levels, and to elevate HDL levels.

Nicotinic acid raises HDL cholesterol and transforms small LDL into the less harmful, normal-sized LDL cholesterol. Niacin therapy moderately reduces LDL cholesterol levels. Among all the pharmaceutical choices, nicotinic acid is the most effective in raising HDL cholesterol. Niacin therapy is also the most effective medication for reducing levels of Lp(a).

Types and Usage

Niacin formulations come in three categories: immediate release, short-term or intermediate release, and sustained or slow-acting release. If you are a candidate for niacin therapy, your physician will determine what formulation is most suitable for you. Most physicians start patients on a low dose and work up to a daily dose of 1.5 to 3 grams. This improves the body's acceptance of the drug.

Another important consideration among different products is the quality of the niacin and the amount that will be absorbed by the body. A challenge with many over-the-counter supplements is that they are prepared in forms that do not break down easily in the digestive system. They essentially pass through the body, without allowing for absorption of any nutrients. Supplements are not regulated by the FDA and are therefore not guaranteed to provide what is shown on the labels.

Niaspan, produced by KOS Pharmaceuticals, is specially formulated and packaged in a way that makes it clear how to regulate the levels of niacin in the bloodstream. Nicotinamide is another form of niacin; however, it is not effective in lowering cholesterol levels.

Side Effects

The challenge with niacin treatment is tolerability. Flushing or hot flashes and itching, the result of the opening of blood vessels, are the most common side effects. If you titrate the drugs appropriately, however, the side effects should decrease over time as your body becomes more tolerant of the therapy. Taking niacin during or after meals, or using aspirin or other additional medications recommended by your physician, can also decrease flushing.

Other side effects include gastrointestinal upset such as nausea, indigestion, gas, vomiting, diarrhea, and even peptic ulcers. More serious risks include liver problems, gout, and high blood sugar. These risks increase as the dosage level is increased.

People who take high blood pressure medications also need to exercise caution with niacin therapy. Taking niacin can amplify the effects of blood pressure medications. People with diabetes typically do not receive niacin therapy because of its effect on blood sugar.

90. Learn about Fibrates

Physicians prescribe fibrates, or fibric acid derivatives, primarily to reduce triglycerides but also to increase HDL cholesterol. Fibrates, however, do not consistently lower LDL cholesterol. Since LDL reduction is usually the primary target of therapy, fibrates are not typically physicians' drug of choice for individuals with elevated cholesterol levels. Even so, you should evaluate the relevance of fibrate therapy to your individual case, since it may be beneficial depending upon your lipid profile.

Fibrate therapy is a treatment option for people with coronary artery disease (CAD) who have low LDL cholesterol but who still have unhealthy lipid levels. Physicians may prescribe fibrates along with statins for people who have both high levels of LDL cholesterol and unhealthy lipid levels. If you are considering drug therapy, be sure to ask your physician whether fibrates are an option.

Types and Usage

Gemfibrozil and fenofibrate are types of fibrates, known by the brand names Lopid and Tricor, respectively. Clofibrate is the third fibrate available in the United States. People on fibrate therapy typically take a dose twice daily, usually thirty minutes before their morning and evening meals.

Side Effects

Most people do not suffer any adverse side effects from fibrate therapy. Some people, however, do experience gastrointestinal problems or headache, dizziness, blurred vision, runny nose, fatigue, or flushing. For some people, fibrates increase the chances of developing gallstones. Tell your health care provider right away about any side effects, particularly if you experience muscle or joint pain or weakness.

91. Follow Tips for Success with Medications

One of the most important things that you can do to help you to stay on your medication program is to understand exactly what type of medication you are taking and why it is best for a person in your condition. This requires you to take some initiative to educate yourself about your lipid profile, your lipid goals, and your dosage schedule. Ask your health care provider the following questions:

- What is my lipid profile and what is my goal of therapy?
- What type of medication (statin, nicotinic acid, fibrate) am I taking?
- Why is that medication best for a person in my condition?
- Are there any food/drug combinations that I should avoid?
- When should I take the medicine and should it be taken with, before, or after meals?
- What should I do if I forget to take a dose?
- What are the side effects of the medication?
- Who should I contact and how in case I have negative side effects?

Being consistent is essential to get the most out of your therapeutic program. Do not change your dosage amount or schedule or quit taking prescription medications without consulting your physician. If you have a hard time with consistency, try some of the following tips:

- Take your medicine at the same time each day.
- Take your medicine when you perform a specific daily act, such as before you brush your teeth.
- Set your watch alarm as a pill reminder.
- Use a pill box that holds each day's prescription in its respective compartment.

- Write yourself a note in a prominent place.
- Write prescription renewal notes in your calendar to remind you before prescriptions run out.

If none of these tips help, consult with your pharmacist for more ideas. Work together with your health care provider as a team. Be sure to observe your reactions to the medication. Take notes, and report everything back to your physician. Keep your follow-up appointments so you can discuss how things are going. Bring your observation notes to your appointment to remind you of things you may easily forget. Bring your prescription bottles as well.

PART VII

SPECIAL CASES

CHAPTER 19

Diabetes and the Metabolic Syndrome

People with diabetes are at higher risk for heart disease than nondiabetics. People who have a cluster of metabolic disorders, characterized as the metabolic syndrome, are also at greater risk for heart disease. The underlying condition—insulin resistance—is present in both conditions but in varying degrees of severity. This chapter provides an overview of the characteristics of these metabolic disorders as well as advice on restoring insulin sensitivity and reducing the associated risks for heart disease and death.

92. Recognize Metabolic Disorders

Metabolic disorders occur when a specific enzyme or cofactor is absent, or is present in insufficient quantities that result in the body's inability to receive particular nutrients. In other words, the body is unable to metabolize foods into nutrients for fuel or to build tissue. For people who have problems producing insulin, which is the key to the uptake of blood glucose (blood sugar), the body is unable to use the glucose that is circulating in the bloodstream for fuel. As a result, blood sugar levels become elevated.

If blood glucose levels are elevated because insulin is not available or insulin resistance is severe, the person is diagnosed with diabetes, which is a metabolic disorder. If, on the other hand, blood glucose levels are elevated because insulin sensitivity is impaired, and this impairment is present with other specific conditions, the person is considered to have a metabolic disorder, described as the "metabolic syndrome." Both of these conditions increase the risk of heart disease. Many people with diabetes, including children and adults, also have lipid disorders, and many also have hypertension. Both of these conditions increase the risk of heart disease. Therefore, not only do people with diabetes need to manage their blood sugar, but it is also important for them to manage their blood pressure and cholesterol carefully.

93. Understand Diabetes

When you eat food that is rich in carbohydrates, such as bread, cereal, or grains, your body breaks it down into glucose. Also referred to as blood sugar, glucose can be used by your body for energy. In a normally functioning system, a healthy pancreas releases insulin into the bloodstream, and this insulin helps to remove the glucose from your bloodstream for your cells to use as fuel. In people who have diabetes, this process is dysfunctional. Either their bodies do not produce any insulin or the insulin that they produce cannot be used.

Because their bodies cannot convert the sugar in the blood into energy, people with diabetes have high levels of glucose in their bloodstream. The kidneys of diabetic people need to work extra hard to filter the blood to remove the excess glucose. This causes frequent urination and excessive thirst from fluid loss.

The liver is also involved in the process of maintaining normal blood sugar levels. After you eat, the sugars from the food enter your bloodstream and are available as fuel, along with the triglycerides. If not all the sugar fuel is used, either due to poor processing based on low insulin or a reduced need for energy based on a low activity level, the liver removes the excess sugar from the bloodstream, much in the same manner as it removes excess cholesterol, and stores it in the liver as glycogen. If for some reason you are unable to eat, the liver later can release this stored glucose into the bloodstream to provide an energy boost. This helps to keep your blood sugar levels in a more constant range.

Type 1 Diabetes

Type 1 diabetes is an autoimmune condition that occurs most often in children and adults younger than age thirty. It is also called juvenile-onset diabetes or insulin-dependent diabetes mellitus. This condition occurs when the body does not produce any insulin, so people with this type of diabetes take daily insulin injections. Approximately 5 to 10 percent of people with diabetes have Type 1. Young people with diabetes are not likely to have heart disease in their youth. As they age, however, their risk of heart disease is greater than the risk to those who do not have diabetes.

Type 2 Diabetes

Type 2 is the most common form of diabetes. It affects about 95 percent of people who have diabetes. This type of diabetes is referred to as maturity-onset diabetes, adult-onset diabetes, or non-insulin-dependent diabetes mellitus.

Type 2 diabetes is a metabolic disorder. In this case, the pancreas produces some insulin but not enough to allow the sugar to enter the body's cells. At the same time, muscle and tissue cells develop a resistance to the insulin. Therefore, even though sugar is flowing in the bloodstream, the body's tissues remain "hungry." Scientists still have been unable to identify the exact mechanism for why insulin resistance occurs, but it seems to have a relationship to excess body fat.

Signs and Symptoms

People often disregard the symptoms of diabetes. However, studies indicate that if diabetes is detected early, the likelihood that complications will develop can be reduced. Therefore, it is important to be knowledgeable about the signs and symptoms of diabetes, particularly if you have a family history of this disease. The signs and symptoms of diabetes include the following:

- Frequent urination
- Excessive thirst
- Extreme hunger
- Unusual weight loss
- Increased fatigue
- Irritability

- Numbness or tingling in feet or legs
- Slow-healing cuts or bruises
- Blurry vision

94. Get Tested for Diabetes

You can determine whether you have diabetes by having the levels of glucose in the bloodstream measured. Before you take a test for diabetes, it is recommended that you go without food or drink for at least nine to twelve hours.

A normal result for a fasting glucose test is between 65 and 109 mg/dL. A result that is lower than 65 mg/dL could indicate low blood sugar, also referred to as hypoglycemia. A result that is between 110 to 125 mg/dL could indicate an impaired fasting glucose level, also known as prediabetes. A result that is higher than 126 mg/dL could indicate diabetes. Consult with your physician for further evaluation if your test indicates that you have hypoglycemia, prediabetes, or diabetes.

Types of Tests

To test your blood glucose levels, you can have either a finger-prick fasting blood sugar test or a hemoglobin A1C test. The tests differ in that a finger-prick test provides a measure of your blood sugar at the moment of the test, while the hemoglobin A1C test shows how your blood sugar has been regulated over the past three-month period by analyzing the hemoglobin, instead of simply the sugar levels. In order to establish a diagnosis of diabetes, a hemoglobin A1C test is necessary.

The American Diabetes Association recommends that people with diabetes take the hemoglobin A1C test two to four times a year. The hemoglobin A1C test does not replace daily self-testing but rather provides a method to assess your success with blood sugar management over time. The FDA has approved a home test. Check with your health care provider to see whether it would be appropriate for you.

95. Learn about the Metabolic Syndrome

Experts have named a group of risk factors—excess weight, physical inactivity, and genetic factors—as likely to indicate the metabolic syndrome, a condition closely associated with the metabolic disorder referred to as insulin resistance or Type 2 diabetes. Because these risk factors often occur together, researchers have a difficult time teasing out the specific contributions of each factor to the overall increased risk of heart disease. While the metabolic syndrome is not a risk factor in and of itself, it is considered to enhance the level of risk, particularly when it is present with high cholesterol levels.

Physicians identify metabolic syndrome when three or more of the following conditions are present:

- Abdominal obesity
- Triglyceride level higher than 140 mg/dL
- HDL cholesterol level of less than 40 mg/dL in men
- HDL cholesterol level of less than 50 mg/dL in women
- Blood pressure greater than or equal to 130/85 mmHg
- Fasting glucose greater than 109 mg/dL

Studies suggest that as many as 24 percent of Americans have the metabolic syndrome. In a study conducted at the Heart Disease Prevention Program at the University of California, Irvine, investigators found that the presence of the metabolic syndrome, in the absence of other risk factors, is associated with an increased risk of coronary artery disease (CAD), cardiovascular disease (CVD), and an increased risk of death. This increased risk of CAD and death from CVD is present even if only one or two risk factors for the metabolic syndrome are present. Research into this area continues.

96. Manage Your Diabetes or Metabolic Syndrome

If your doctor diagnoses you with diabetes or you have the metabolic syndrome, it's even more important that you adopt healthy lifestyle habits. When you address the root causes of this condition—excess weight and a sedentary lifestyle—sensitivity to insulin is restored, and the risk factors are reduced. Lifestyle changes can make a huge difference. If you have diabetes, it can be successfully managed. If you are prediabetic, you can avoid becoming diabetic.

The Power of Healthful Eating

Physical activity and healthful eating need to go hand in hand to improve the factors associated with diabetes and the metabolic syndrome. Healthy nutrition should follow the guidelines discussed in Chapter 8, including eating a diet of primarily plant-based foods. Total dietary fat should represent between 25 to 35 percent of total calories, but it should be composed mostly of unsaturated vegetable fats. Researchers note that dietary fat, rather than calories, carbohydrates, or even sugar intake, seems to be a critical factor in

Type 2 diabetes, although researchers have not yet been able to identify the exact mechanisms.

The Power of Exercise

Your exercise program to improve insulin sensitivity should include both heart-pumping cardiovascular activities and strength-training exercises to tone up your muscles. Regular exercise helps you maintain healthy blood sugar levels by burning fuels and by helping you to achieve and maintain a healthy weight and shed excess body fat. Improvements in glucose tolerance and insulin sensitivity are usually short-lived, however, and deteriorate within three days of your last workout. This factor makes regular aerobic exercise vital.

Cardiovascular or aerobic exercise, such as walking, is critically important for managing blood sugar levels and improving your body's ability to use insulin. Try to be active on at least three nonconsecutive days and up to five sessions per week. Ideally, your aerobic exercise session should last at least thirty minutes. It's not necessary to work at a high intensity. Take it easy, and progress gradually. If thirty minutes is too long, start with ten-minute bouts and accumulate thirty minutes in one day.

According to the position taken by the American College of Sports Medicine (ACSM) on exercise and Type 2 diabetes, resistance or weight training has the potential to improve muscle strength and endurance, enhance flexibility and body composition, decrease risk factors for CVD, and result in improved glucose tolerance and insulin sensitivity. Strength training can also increase the resting metabolic rate to assist in weight control. Regular exercise that includes aerobics and strength training also provides important emotional health benefits, including reduced stress, heightened feelings of well-being, and enhanced quality of life.

CHAPTER 20

Special Groups and High Cholesterol

While the same general principles related to healthy nutrition, regular physical activity, no smoking, and weight and stress management apply to all people, there are certain special considerations for people with particular needs. These people include children, teens, and older adults. Women also have needs and special considerations that are distinct from those of men.

97. Learn about High Cholesterol in Children and Adolescents

Recently, medical professionals have been paying greater attention to childhood cholesterol levels as concern rises over the increasing incidence of Type 2 diabetes, inactivity, and overweight issues among kids. Since heart disease is a slow, progressive disease, more and more attention is being given to the significance of healthy habits from youth.

An Inherited Disorder

Children from certain families that include a parent or grandparent who had heart disease at an early age are genetically prone to have high cholesterol levels. If a male relative had a heart attack before age fifty-five or a female relative before age sixty-five, this places a child in a high-risk category.

Just the Facts

Statistics reveal that approximately one in 500 children have inherited hypercholesterolemia. These children have a 50 percent risk of having heart disease before age fifty. If this condition is detected early, children can incorporate healthy habits to greatly reduce their risk of having heart disease.

Guidelines for Blood Lipid Levels

The National Cholesterol Education Program's Expert Panel on Blood Cholesterol in Children and Adolescents recommends these guidelines for cholesterol levels in children and adolescents age two to nineteen: Total cholesterol is acceptable if it is less than 170 mg/dL. It is considered borderline if it is 170 to 199 mg/dL and high if it is 200 mg/dL or greater. LDL cholesterol should ideally be less than 110 mg/dL, with borderline levels ranging from 110 to 129 mg/dL. At levels of 130 or greater, LDL is considered high. The guidelines also recommend that HDL levels should be greater than or equal to 35 mg/dL, and that triglycerides should be less than or equal to 150 mg/dL.

Experts disagree about the role of cholesterol-lowering drugs for children. Government treatment guidelines first recommend lifestyle changes such as first improving eating habits, increasing physical activity, and managing weight.

The American Heart Association and the federal government recommend that cholesterol-lowering drugs be recommended only for those children over ten years of age who have high LDL levels even after changes in diet. Other experts, however, remain concerned about the long-term effectiveness of drug therapy. Medical professionals uniformly recommend healthful lifestyle changes as being of paramount importance for children to enjoy good health.

98. Be Aware of Special Considerations for Teens

Teens, their parents, and health care providers also need to be sensitive to cholesterol issues affecting today's youth. Studies show that between 15 and 20 percent of the population already has atherosclerotic plaque by age twenty. About 10 percent of adolescents between the ages of twelve and nineteen have cholesterol levels that exceed 200 mg/dL. The risk for adolescents is increased further by using oral contraceptives and cigarettes. In one study among females age twelve to seventeen years, researchers found that the total cholesterol of oral contraceptive users was significantly higher than in nonusers. Birth control users who are also smokers are at even higher risk for heart disease.

99. Know the Facts about Women and High Cholesterol

Heart disease is the number-one killer of women. In America, heart diseases kill nearly half a million women per year, more than the next seven causes of death combined, including all forms of cancer. The recommended levels of blood lipids are for the most part the same for women and men; however, women have some distinct differences that merit special consideration.

Silent Heart Disease

Women in particular suffer from "silent heart disease," which often goes undiagnosed. A silent heart attack is a result of atherosclerotic buildup in coronary arteries that causes death of so little heart tissue that it may be symptom-free or easily confused with feelings of indigestion or anxiety.

According to the American Heart Association, clinicians often attribute chest pain in women to other causes. As more and more studies are conducted on women subjects, more information about the differences in the development of heart disease in men and women is becoming available.

Other Concerns for Women

Pregnancy is a time when a woman's lipid profile tends to change. Pregnant women typically have an increase in blood cholesterol levels. This is not cause for alarm, unless otherwise noted by your health care provider.

Also, oral contraception can increase levels of blood cholesterol as well as blood pressure. Smokers, in particular, have a higher risk of heart disease and stroke if they also take birth control pills.

Testing and Research

One more confounding factor in the diagnosis and treatment of heart disease in women is that diagnostic tests and procedures are not as accurate for women as they are for men. For example, an exercise stress test has a higher likelihood of showing a false positive or a false negative for women subjects. More expensive diagnostic tests tend to be more precise. Discuss all your options thoroughly with your health care provider.

100. Understand the Age Factor: Cholesterol and Menopause

A woman's risk of heart disease increases approximately ten to fifteen years later than the average man's. This disparity is reflected in guidelines that state that an age of forty-five or above is a risk factor for a man; for a woman, on the other hand, age does not become a risk factor until she is fifty-five. The reasons for this difference are not fully understood. Some of it is thought to be due to the protective effects of estrogen. A woman's heart disease risk rises when she becomes postmenopausal, regardless of whether menopause occurred naturally or as the result of surgery.

By the time a woman reaches the age of seventy-five or older, her risk of heart attack is approximately the same as that of a man's. Women age seventy-five and above actually have a higher risk of death by stroke than men.

The reasons for this are not clear. Some researchers suggest that it may simply be due to the fact that atherosclerosis is a slow, progressive disease and more women live longer than men. More research on women's health issues is needed to bring further light to these questions.

Another aspect of menopause that may contribute to a woman's higher risk of heart disease is the tendency to gain weight, particularly around the abdominal area. Abdominal fat that creates an apple-shaped physique is known to be a sign for increased risk of heart disease.

101. Maintain Healthy Habits as You Age

Most deaths from heart disease occur in the older adult population. Men age sixty-five and above and women age seventy-five and above are classified as older adults for the purpose of discussing heart disease.

One study among older adults with an average age of seventy-two showed that eating fatty fish at least once a week reduced the risk of heart attack by as much as 44 percent. Clearly, life extension can even occur at older ages. Quality of life is also important and can be maintained through healthy nutrition, regular physical activity, and weight management. Even studies of people over the age of ninety showed that strength training with weights could bring improvements.

A lifetime of healthy habits is always the ideal situation. But few of us live ideal lives. We can all make daily life more pleasurable by enhancing health, which includes maintaining healthy lipid levels. It is never too late to take steps to improve your quality of life.

Index